'Lizaveta van Munsteren's new study provides important new insights. This thoughtful, well researched book will interest anyone concerned with the history of 'the talking cure', and the politics of the human sciences in the Soviet empire.'

**Daniel Pick**, *professor emeritus, Birkbeck, University of London; training analyst, the British Psychoanalytical Society*

'This comprehensive and thorough study by Lizaveta van Munsteren illustrates how Freudian ideas were denied and removed in the Soviet Union. The book then effectively describes the 'return of the repressed'. Psychoanalysis re-emerged in the work of great and unforgettable figures in the history of Soviet psychology.'

**Alberto Angelini**, *psychoanalyst, Sapienza University, National Film School (CSC), Rome, Italy*

# The Vicissitudes of Psychoanalysis in Soviet Russia, 1930–1980

This book considers the changing fortunes of psychoanalysis in Soviet Russia from 1930 to 1980.

Approaching social history in a psychoanalytic key, Lizaveta van Munsteren argues that the growing split between official and informal languages of the time produced multiple strategies to keep alive the conversation around prohibited subjects. Through original archival research on figures such as Bluma Zeigarnik, Alexander Luria, Filipp Bassin and Dmitry Uznadze, van Munsteren offers a more nuanced understanding of Soviet studies of the unconscious and the role of language in the formation of the mind and in mental disturbances. This book makes a significant contribution to the historiography of psychoanalysis and to the study of the cultural influence of psychoanalysis and its interdisciplinary engagements.

*The Vicissitudes of Psychoanalysis in Soviet Russia, 1930–1980* will appeal to historians of psychoanalysis and psychology in Soviet Russia, psychosocial researchers and anyone interested in the critical history of psychoanalysis.

**Lizaveta van Munsteren**, PhD, is a clinician and academic with a long-standing interest in psychoanalytic theory and history. She is currently a post-doctoral researcher with the FREEPSY project at the University of Essex, working on theoretical formulations of the psychoanalytic frame in free clinics, and archives of free clinics in Vienna and Budapest.

History of Psychoanalysis

Series Editor Peter L. Rudnytsky

This series seeks to present outstanding new books that illuminate any aspect of the history of psychoanalysis from its earliest days to the present, and to reintroduce classic texts to contemporary readers.

**Theories and Practices of Psychoanalysis in Central Europe**
Narrative Assemblages of Self Analysis, Life Writing, and Fiction
*Agnieszka Sobolewska*

**Sigmund Freud and his Patient Margarethe Csonka**
A Case of Homosexuality in a Woman in Modern Vienna
*Michal Shapira*

**Sigmund Freud, 1856-1939**
A Biographical Compendium
*Christfried Toegel*

**The Marquis de Puysegur and Artificial Somnambulism**
Memoirs to Contribute to the History and Establishment of Animal Magnetism
*Edited and translated by Adam Crabtree and Sarah Osei-Bonsu*

**The Subversive Edge of Psychoanalysis**
*David James Fisher*

**Freud's British Family**
Reclaiming Lost Lives in Manchester and London
*Roger Willoughby*

For further information about this series please visit https://www.routledge.com/The-History-of-Psychoanalysis-Series/book-series/KARNHIPSY

# The Vicissitudes of Psychoanalysis in Soviet Russia, 1930–1980

Lizaveta van Munsteren

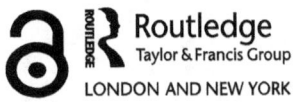
LONDON AND NEW YORK

Designed cover image: Getty Images

First published 2026
by Routledge
4 Park Square, Milton Park, Abingdon, Oxon OX14 4RN

and by Routledge
605 Third Avenue, New York, NY 10158

*Routledge is an imprint of the Taylor & Francis Group, an informa business*

© 2026 Lizaveta van Munsteren

The right of Lizaveta van Munsteren to be identified as author of this work has been asserted in accordance with sections 77 and 78 of the Copyright, Designs and Patents Act 1988.

This publication was supported by the University of Essex's open access fund.

The Open Access version of this book, available at www.taylorfrancis.com, has been made available under a Creative Commons [Creative Commons Attribution-No Derivatives 4.0 International (CC-BY-ND)] 4.0 International license.

Any third party material in this book is not included in the OA Creative Commons license, unless indicated otherwise in a credit line to the material. Please direct any permissions enquiries to the original rightsholder.

*Trademark notice*: Product or corporate names may be trademarks or registered trademarks, and are used only for identification and explanation without intent to infringe.

*British Library Cataloguing-in-Publication Data*
A catalogue record for this book is available from the British Library

*Library of Congress Cataloging-in-Publication Data*
A catalog record has been requested for this book

ISBN: 978-1-032-86376-4 (hbk)
ISBN: 978-1-032-84593-7 (pbk)
ISBN: 978-1-003-52726-8 (ebk)

DOI: 10.4324/9781003527268

Typeset in Times New Roman
by Taylor & Francis Books

# Contents

|   |   |   |
|---|---|---|
| | *List of figures* | viii |
| | *To my reader* | ix |
| | *Acknowledgements* | x |
| | *A note on names and translations* | xi |
| | *Abbreviations and glossary* | xii |
| | Introduction | 1 |
| 1 | Histories of psychoanalysis in Soviet Russia and its discontents | 22 |
| 2 | Freud in the public discourse | 60 |
| 3 | Zeigarnik, Luria and Vygotsky: Building pathopsychology | 81 |
| 4 | Luria's turn to psychophysiology, language and consciousness | 107 |
| 5 | The Soviet unconscious: Uznadze, Bassin and others | 129 |
| | Epilogue | 164 |
| | *References* | 167 |
| | *Index* | 178 |

# Figure

4.1 Psychological schema of the word concept (Freud, 1891)   122

# To my reader

In his work on the unconscious, Wilfred Bion summarises several points about the impossibility for the conscious to grasp the unconscious, hence the impossibility of the linear way to capture the latter. The unconscious is a multidimensional phenomenon, which only reveals itself clearly while we are in the dream. When waking up, we lose the 'wholeness' of the picture and clarity of it and only can deliver a dream in patches. Our consciousness works like a sewing machine, putting pieces together in a coherent blanket of a story we can tell.

While my research is not directly a study of the unconscious of the individual, it is still trying to catch something invisible: in Soviet society, in texts, in ideas. It attempts to read between the lines and to capture processes that emerged in the dimension of unspoken. Thus, I was faced with the difficulty of putting into words something that by its nature exists outside of the verbal register. Simultaneously, this research is a work of translation, first of all, because English is my second language, and the work you are reading was proofread and corrected by multiple editors who corrected it for the English reader to make it stylistically coherent and grammatically correct. Second, materials and ideas for this research were translated from Russian and inevitably lost some of their complexity because the translation of meaning reduces the unspoken cultural addition that every text holds.

When writing this book, I was careful about how to put the pieces of my research and ideas together. However, at some point, I realized that they cannot be told as a whole story. Many of the facts and events described below must be combined by the reader's mind to make sense, so when reading this book, please allow the gaps and uncertainties not to be resolved immediately by my voice telling you what to think. Only after reading certain chapters will previous chapters will make more sense and I hope that, after finishing the last chapter, you will return to the beginning with more understanding of what it was all about.

As much as I wanted to make this research comprehensive, this work is incomplete.

# Acknowledgements

This book is based on research that at various times was supported and supervised by Sarah Marks, Stephen Frosh and Brendan McGeever, whose guidance and expertise set up the excellence bar I only occasionally reach. Without my mother, who went to enquire at GARF archives in Moscow on my behalf amid the pandemic, this work would not have relied on archival materials. My colleagues in FREEPSY at the University of Essex, Ana Minozzo, Ana Tomcic and especially Raluca Soreanu facilitated this book to emerge.

The earlier version of Chapter 3 was published as an article in 2023: 'Bluma Zeigarnik: A Missing Name in the History of Psychoanalysis in Soviet Russia?' *Psychoanalysis and History*, 25(1), 31–58 https://doi.org/10.3366/pah.2023.0451

I am grateful to the Journal for permission to use it, also, to the editor Matt ffytche, and anonymous reviewers, and especially reviewer 1 whose comments and suggestions helped make my work on Zeigarnik sound.

I am endlessly grateful to my dearest Gustavo Sánchez, Alexander Kravtsov, Anna Svarovskaya and Lena Kostyleva, whose intellect and humour kept me sane, and who were always there for me. I am very grateful to my colleagues in various institutions who at different times contributed with discussions or readings of various parts of my work, Francis Hornyold-Strickland, Evan Sedgwick-Jell, Anna Shadrina, Elena Gkivisi, Daniel Gilsenan, Megan Williams, Helen Wessels, Martin Wagner. And most of all my husband Eric, whose skills of making coffee and creating space for me while I was writing were invaluable for this work to be finished.

I dedicate this work to my father, who will never read it, but whose generosity and love in the past made this book possible to be written today.

# A note on names and translations

I use the Library of Congress system of transliteration, except when author's name has been published using a different system (for example, Vygotsky, not Vygotskii). For cities in Ukraine, I have transliterated from Ukrainian spelling (Kyiv, not Kiev). All translations from Russian-language sources are my own.

# Abbreviations and glossary

| | |
|---|---|
| AMS | Academy of Medical Sciences |
| GARF | State Archive of the Russian Federation |
| MSU | Moscow State University |
| Narkom | People's Commissariat |
| Narkompros | People's Commissariat for Education |
| Politizdat | Political Literature Publishing House |
| RAMN | Russian Academy of Medical Sciences |
| RAN | Russian Academy of Sciences |
| Uchpedgiz | State Publishing House of Student and Pedagogical Literature |
| VAK | Higher Attestation Commission |
| VKP(b) | The All-Union Communist Party (of Bolsheviks) |
| blat | A colloquial term to denote ways of getting things done through personal contacts, associated with using connections, pulling strings and exchanging favours. |
| novyi byt | 'New way of living', a Soviet campaign in the 1920s aimed at developing new habits, practices and customs for domestic life based on communist ideals. |
| kulturnost | 'Cultureness', in the 1930s referred to the practices of good manners, personal hygiene, dressing, level of literacy, education and knowledge of communist ideology etc. which were promoted in Soviet society to adapt peasants to becoming 'cultural' citizens of the new society. |
| kommunalka | Communal apartment in which several unrelated families or individuals lived in isolated living rooms and shared communal areas such as kitchen, bathroom and toilet. |

# Introduction

"If you really, really want something, but it is prohibited, then it's allowed" (my grandmother)

## Part 1: 1958

An event that will become central point of insight for this book occurred in Moscow in 1958.

The event was titled *The Scientific Meeting on the Problem of the Ideological Struggle Against Contemporary Freudism* [*Nauchnoe Soveshchanie po Voprosam Ideologicheskoi Bor'by s Sovremennym Freidizmom*][1] and it was held under the initiative of the Presidium of the Academy of Medical Sciences of USSR, further called the Freud Session.

The format of the *scientific sessions* was quite common in the practice of this period and was structured in the same way as the Party sessions. Prominent academics in the field gathered for a discussion on the chosen problem. Normally it would end with a resolution or a plan of action on how to solve it. The best-known scientific session in psychiatry, physiology and psychology was the *Pavlov Session*, held in 1950–1951. The Pavlov Session was a turning point for the psy-disciplines and aimed to eradicate idealistic and bourgeois theories that were still serving as a groundwork for Soviet scientists. It resulted in the major turn to Pavlovian physiology for studies on the human and excluded the possibility of psychological explanations of the mind, including psychoanalytic ideas. The effect of this session lasted until 1962 when the *All-Union Conference on Philosophical Issues in the Physiology of Higher Nervous Activity and Psychology* [*Vsesoiuznaia Konferentsiia po Filosofskim Voprosam Fiziologii Vysshei Nervnoi Deiatel'nosti i Psikhologii*] rejected the monopoly of Pavlov's theories in the field and officially brought back psychological theories.

In this context, the session dedicated to the struggle against Freudism in 1958 did not quite fit the course given during the Pavlov Session and raises questions about its objective.

DOI: 10.4324/9781003527268-1

This chapter has been made available under a CC-BY-ND 4.0 license.

Everything about this session was unusual. It was dedicated to the discussion of Freud and his ideas, their place in the scientific world and the role that Soviet scientists should play in addressing the critique of psychoanalysis. If we follow the existing historical narrative, psychoanalysis was 'banned' in the 1930s and, after the Pavlov Session and the turn of Soviet psychology to physiology, the last leftovers of psychoanalysis should have been eradicated by the 1950s. Yet, the Freud Session happened. Was it organized as a reminder not to follow Freud after 28 years of an official 'ban' and an eight-year legacy of Pavlovian domination of the field? Or was it a gesture of loyalty and reassurance that Soviet scientists were still on track with Pavlov?

In the broad context of the time, these questions relate to the overall place of Freud, psychoanalysis and Freudism in the Soviet Union in the years 1930–1980. What were the vicissitudes of psychoanalysis in psychology and psychiatry, the disciplines that were the first to pick up psychoanalytic ideas upon their arrival in 1903? What was the destiny of Freud's heritage among other disciplines? Were there any other interested readers of Freud in the Soviet Union during this period? What did pre-revolutionary followers of Freud make of his ideas in the later years of their work under Soviet rule?

A historical clue has the potential to answer these questions. The Freud Session happened in a period of de-Stalinization, which introduced a window for the revision of Stalinist policies. From that angle it appears as an attempt to bring back discussion about Freud, whose name had been prohibited from mention since the 1930s. But what kept psychoanalysis present in the academic discussion before, if anything? Between 1930 and 1958 there were a good 28 years.

We have only partial answers to these questions. The amount of research on the history of psychoanalysis in Russia remains relatively small and was mostly conducted more than 20 years ago. A study by Alex Kozulin (1984) explores the professional establishment of early Russian and Soviet psychologists, and their turn to psychoanalysis and against it, as well as early attempts to combine psychoanalysis with Marxism. It focuses on several names engaged with psychoanalysis and their personal histories. Elisabeth Roudinesco (1990) reflects on the destiny of psychoanalysis in Soviet times due to the ideological shift in science as a whole. Alexander Etkind's (1997) pioneer study of the relationship between psychoanalysis and Russians is a rich detective story of personal interconnections of early psychoanalytic enthusiasts. It focuses on the impossibility of the development of psychoanalysis under Soviet rule due its ideological incompatibility and clashes with politics. It stops in 1930. Martin Miller (1998) covers the whole period of the USSR as a very detailed story of the sequence of events around psychoanalysis. His focus is on the establishment of institutions and organizations around psychoanalysis, as well as major responses to psychoanalytic ideas within scientific society. Alberto Angelini (1988, 2008) searches for an answer as to why psychoanalysis was destined to be repressed in the Soviet Union. Dmitrii Rozhdestvenskii (2009) analyses why a Russian 'soul' with all its openness to self-reflection did not hold to the psychoanalytic method and why the early psychoanalytic movement 'failed'. More recent research by Hanna Proctor (2020) touches on the history of two figures of the early psychoanalytic movement in Russia – Alexander Luria and Lev Vygotsky – and their attempts to combine psychoanalysis with some experimental techniques as well as to engage psychoanalysis with Marxism.

The studies listed above shaped not only the knowledge of psychoanalysis in this period, but also the narrative of it. The 'official' story, found in all above texts, in short, says that psychoanalysis arrived in Russia in 1900, flourished in the 1920s, was banned in the 1930s, started to re-appear again in the late 1980s and was rehabilitated in the 1990s, together with post-Freudian Western theories. According to this timeline, for 50 years psychoanalysis disappeared from scientific discussion. The fact that the same sequence of events is told the same way in different research suggests that later scholars inherited the views of the previous generation without ever subjecting these accounts to scrutiny. Sometimes, in order to support the established narrative, the socio-historical context was abandoned. For example, Rozhdestvenskii (2009) writes that after the 1930s members of the early psychoanalytic movement left it and 'simply trained for a new profession'. Considering the fact that in the 1930s for supporting psychoanalysis one can easily become an enemy of the state and get killed for anti-state views, for early enthusiasts of psychoanalysis to train for a new profession might have been a life-saving decision, not simply a choice.

Yes, the development of psychoanalytic institutions was discontinued between 1930 and 1980, as was the publication of the works of Freud and other psychoanalysts, with several exceptions. It was no longer easy to obtain books on psychoanalysis; they were available in the libraries for those readers who had a special permission pass. Freud's name continued to circulate in the public press and academic literature, even if under the sauce of criticism.

Does this mean psychoanalysis was not used as a theory at all? Does it mean psychoanalysis was not practised clinically, or that it did not influence other clinical practices? What happened to the early enthusiasts of psychoanalysis, and where did their interest in psychoanalysis lead them? Were there new readers of Freud during this period of 50 years and how did they make use of psychoanalysis? My book seeks, if not to answer these questions fully, then at least to attempt to find them.

But let us return to the meaning of the Freud Session in 1958, an event important for its potential to give us some research clues. When I initially approached the topic, my focus was on several prominent names that were associated with psychoanalysis (or at least mentioned in the existing literature): Alexander Luria, Filipp Bassin, Dmitry Uznadze. Reading around the topic very soon brought me to the Freud Session. I was already familiar with a lot of fragments of pre-Revolutionary enthusiasm for psychoanalysis and the struggle of the 1930s due to political turbulence. I could not make much sense at that time of what I was seeing in the literature having more questions than answers, all around the Freud Session. The shift in my vision occurred, however, not in the library, but in the Everyman Cinema in Maida Vale. I went to the cinema to clear my head from research questions and to watch *Men in Black: International* (2019) – a blockbuster comedy that promises flashing images, extended fighting scenes and minimal dialogue. But instead of thoughtless fun, I got a revelation.

Throughout the film, I found myself relating to the feelings of the heroine, Agent M. During the movie she was continuously asking Agent H about a specific event in the past, and he kept repeating the story of what happened in literally the same sequence of words. Dissatisfied, she asked him again and again, hoping to hear some additional details. Instead, she only received the same X-Y-Z answer. At some point, she reached the peak of annoyance and curiosity and was about to abandon her investigation. She was puzzled and ready to drop it, and I knew exactly how she felt. I felt the same! That scene echoed the continuous feeling of dissatisfaction I had in my attempt to find answers to questions about psychoanalysis in Soviet Russia in the existing literature. Something was missing in the description of events, during the period spanning 1930–1980, and my mind could not make sense of it. Moreover, the literature did not explain why some of these events even happened!

Of course, the level of precision in a historical narrative is limited by the availability of evidence like documents, artefacts, stories around the event, etc. Normally we would have at least two versions or not exactly similar accounts, showing that the same facts might be interpreted in different ways. The absence of differences in how history was written across texts that I read was one of the recurrent themes of my puzzle.

If I followed the narrative of the disappearance of psychoanalysis after 1930, I could not find an explanation for the Symposium on the Unconscious that took place in 1979, where 1,400 participants, Soviet and Western psychiatrists, physiologists, psychologists, linguists, and philosophers gathered for several days in Tbilisi, Georgian SSR. It did not explain pieces of research on the nature of unconscious activity undertaken by several Soviet scientists such as Uznadze, Anokhin, and Bernstein between 1930 and 1960. It did not explain the study on affects and the nature of aphasia so close to Freudian, conducted by Luria and his school in the 1940s. It did not explain the development of an approach to schizophrenia, based on the importance of language with lots of resemblances of psychoanalytic theory, invented by Zeigarnik and her colleagues in the 1930s. It did not explain that even in general therapy, a long conversation with the patient as a necessary part of the treatment became standard and such terms as "internal picture of illness" and "iatrogenic diseases"[2] appeared.[3] How did such attention to mental functioning and unconscious phenomena happen in Soviet science between 1930 and 1980 if psychoanalysis had completely vanished and was replaced by Pavlovian reflexology?

Yes, Soviet scientists might not have been psychoanalysts in the conventional sense, upholding a tradition of training. However, what if Soviet scientists in their own ways succeeded in following and expanding upon Freud's ideas?

But let's go back to the repetition, which puzzled Agent M in the movie. Eventually, she and Agent H both realized that the repetition occurred because his memory was erased by a machine widely used by Men in Black. When something extraordinary happened with ordinary people or they saw something they should not have seen, like aliens, Men in Black used the eraser to keep the lives of ordinary people contained, but they never used the machine against each other. This machine not only erased the memory but replaced it by made-up memory, concentrated in one cover phrase, pronounced by the agent. And this phrase was exactly what Agent H kept repeating! That is why he was not able to add any details to it. For them, that discovery helped to uncover treason in the agency. For me, that discovery mirrored the repetition I had been dealing with. It was a reiteration of the same story about the ban of psychoanalysis, the dissolution of the psychoanalytic society, the abandonment of psychoanalytic ideas by former enthusiasts in 1930–1980. And if, for the film's protagonists, it was 'a happy ending', for me it marked a happy beginning, and a shift in how I looked at my findings.

There I immediately thought of the repetition phenomena described by Sigmund Freud in *The Interpretation of Dreams* (1900). When talking to a patient about the dream and attempting interpretation, he suggests psychoanalysts ask patients during the session to repeat the dream straight away after it's been told. And while a patient is repeating it, the analyst should look for the gaps or episodes of changes, where the plot alters. Freud argues that those moments of a difference reveal the truth of the unconscious. He explains that when a dream is repeated in the exact same way, the strong work of the patient's conscious censorship becomes evident. That means that the work of the patient's conscious defence has already been done and the primary unconscious material is censored. Freud calls it the secondary revision process. Moments of inconsistency, on the other hand, are moments of truth, where unconscious ideas break through the censorship.

While reading for my research, which always led me to new sources, I needed the way out of the same history repeated again and again. It seemed as if the censorship worked so well it was impossible to get to the hidden material. With the knowledge about the success of Agent M, I waited for my own break through the repetition pattern. The moment of enlightenment happened when, for the third time, I encountered a description of the event held in 1958 in Moscow, at the Freud Session. For the first time, I came across an analysis of this event in Miller's study but didn't see much importance in it. Then I read about it in the article of Angelini, and only after that, did I read the original piece. Coming back to Miller's writing again made me realize that my reading was different! It seemed like I managed to get through the censorship and discover something new – something not yet shaped by an analysis I had read at that time.

So, what happened in 1958? From the position of Miller, it was a session dedicated to the criticism of psychoanalysis. This session represented how strong the criticism of Freud was, and how solid was the position of Pavlov in Soviet academia. Also, Soviet scientists were not really up to date on psychoanalytic theories, and in their criticism, we see a lot of misunderstanding of the basic concepts of psychoanalysis (Miller, 1998). How did Angelini see this event? He says, "On this occasion the usual range of neurological, psychological and philosophical criticisms of psychoanalytic theory was re-affirmed" (Angelini, 2008, p. 378) – his focus is in agreement with Miller's view.

However, Angelini continues, "the influence of Freudian thought had started to be felt, in both scientific and cultural contexts" (Angelini, 2008, p. 378). The idea of the influence is supported by the fact that "the scholars, V.N. Miasishchev and P.K. Anokhin, claimed that, in order to be able to criticize psychoanalysis, it was necessary to study it in depth" (p. 378). Although this is almost everything Angelini mentions about that event in 1958, it is important because Anokhin, a well-known physiologist and author of the Theory of Functional Systems, at that time was already on my list of scientists who applied ideas about the unconscious in physiology. In the article on this event in Russian, we find his argument: "The brain does not function as a screen, that responds only" to the external reality, but "captures a certain amount of impressions that are outside the realm of consciousness" (Ovcharenko, 1999, p. 115). Miller and Angelini described Miasishchev as someone who referred to Freud indirectly and used psychoanalytic ideas in his clinical practice (Angelini, 2008, p. 377). Miasishchev called the theory he invented the psychology of relations, and it appears as a revised version of psychoanalysis, without reference to psychoanalysis. It became apparent that this period of Soviet history may contain much more evidence of the presence of psychoanalysis, and interest in psychoanalysis, than has previously been expressed.

Holding to these clues, I attempted to reconstruct a different story. That's why this book turned to what we can call an extended notion of the archive and memory. For the possibility of a more nuanced reading, I tried to engage with as much material as I could find. I included in the scope the periodic press of that time to see if there were any mentions of Freud or psychoanalysis, both public and academic. I closely read all of the books and monographs from the period 1930–1980 that touch on psychology, neurology and physiology that I could find. Most of the primary sources – articles and monographs written by Zeigarnik, Luria, Bassin, and Uznadze, archival documents, publications in the scientific journals and public press I used for this research are in Russian. Some of them I use in parallel with their published English translations; most of the translations from Russian are done by me.

This book borrows a lot from the social and political history of Soviet Russia to better understand the context in which the lives of academics I read were situated. In the book you will see how former followers of psychoanalysis endured the worsening conditions of the Soviet regime that impacted their lives, the science, and the society they lived in. For those who lived through 1930–1980: Zeigarnik, Luria, Bassin, as we have seen, research conditions changed dramatically so they had to alter their work. For Vygotsky and Uznadze, who died in 1935 and 1950 respectively, that meant the alteration of their ideas by others.

I wrote this book during the Ukraine war, grappling with devastation and uncertainty about how to address the pressing political issues of both the past and present. The Russian imperialist ambitions, the internal Russification policies within the USSR, and the complex relationships between Soviet Republics, both during the Soviet era and after its collapse, all played a role in shaping the trajectory of psychoanalysis during the period discussed in this book. As you will discover, these dynamics were evident well before Russia's attack on Ukraine but often remained obscured and rarely openly discussed.

The centralization of academia and accumulation of resources in the capital forced scientific migration, hence a lot of events in this book happened in Soviet Moscow. Geography of origins is very diverse, and none of the figures of this book were, in fact, Russians. Luria came from Tatar ASSR, Zeigarnik from Lithuanian SSR, Vygotsky was from Belarusian SSR, Bassin was from Ukrainian SSR and Uznadze from Georgian SSR. Except for Uznadze all were of Jewish descent.

I chose the years 1930–1980 not only because they are known as the times of the 'ban' or repression of psychoanalysis – it is important to have such a wide period to bring into the entanglement of an older generation of psychologists who were in the vanguard of psychoanalysis and a new generation of psychologists who were born in the period of 'critical' views on psychoanalysis without understanding the roots of their teachers, and nevertheless continued a dialogue with psychoanalysis.

As many revisionists of the history of Soviet science discovered, the worsening of conditions did not necessarily lead to the worsening of the quality of ideas or the research produced. The same applies to my discoveries. We don't know, of course, what their career path would have looked like if not for the Soviet regime, and how their ideas could have been transformed, but we can see that despite the need to shift their research, they kept certain ideas intact while at the same time being changed. At the end of this research, I remain curious over whether their interest in psychoanalytic theory provided them with the resources to manage these vicissitudes. And also, I am wondering, is it possible to preserve psychoanalytic theory and change it at the same time?

Situated between institutional psychoanalysts who recognize psychoanalysis solely through the lens of institutional history and Russian academia – which, for various reasons, struggles to acknowledge psychoanalysis within the theoretical contributions of Soviet scientists – this book aims to contribute to issues beyond regional boundaries. The debate over whether the historiography of psychoanalysis should be confined to the history of its prominent figures and institutions has been ongoing for some time. Increasing attention is now being given to the histories of those on the periphery and margins, ordinary men and women whose practices and ideas contributed to the development of psychoanalysis without claiming the status of revisionists or pioneers of new psychoanalytic schools.

This is why histories of suffering, loss and struggle are important for my book. Not only because the atrocities of the Soviet times that are well known and recorded by many historians constituted the reality in which all the participants of my book lived and worked in. Also, because this book would like to contribute in turning the history of psychoanalysis away from the polished story of great achievements and thoughts.

This book offers a series of interventions into known histories, and it does not pursue a comprehensive account on Bluma Zeigarnik, Alexander Luria, Filipp Bassin or Dmitry Uznadze. Rather, it aims to nuance and accentuate their histories considering the assumption of not a complete disappearance of psychoanalysis from their work as well. I argue that instead of being repressed, psychoanalysis in Soviet Russia was negated. In the result of the Russification and anti-bourgeoise campaign references to Freud were either erased or turned into 'critique', and only with the work of negation psychoanalytic ideas could be mentioned. That allowed in some shape and form for it to be used for thinking in other disciplines, but never in the form that could be recognized as an institute.

After I wrote this book it became apparent to me, that one of the main curiosities I had was to try to understand the minds and thinking processes of people who were forced to live under ideological pressure and to consider their strategies of survival, especially when related to the question of dignity and identity.

Chapter 1 begins with a more detailed introduction of the current historical narrative of the acceptance and disappearance of psychoanalysis in Russia before the Revolution of 1917 and in the Soviet times. It picks up the threads of engagement with Marxist ideas and clinical developments that psychoanalysis received upon its arrival. It traces general shifts in Soviet science such as Russification and ideological alignment, as well as specific to psychology and psychiatry shift to physiology and exclusion of social reasoning from the scope of theories and clinical methods. The chapter proposes the idea that after the peak of political repressions in the 1930s, discussion of psychoanalysis was not repressed or driven underground but was covered by the disguise of negation. It suggests that following shifts in language, that occurred on all levels in Soviet society of that time, enthusiasts of psychoanalysis had to learn to 'speak Soviet' to continue the conversation around it. It concludes that with the inclusion of social strategies and informal practices that emerged in the Soviet society the historiography of psychoanalysis can turn to the re-interpretation and more nuanced reading of Freud Session in 1958. Also, the idea of negation of psychoanalysis as a disguised strategy opens the space to see the work of Luria, Zeigarnik, Bassin and Uznadze, which is going to be discussed in further chapters, as examples of productive interdisciplinary elaboration of the psychoanalytic theory.

Chapter 2 continues to research the effects of language and ideological shifts in Soviet society and turns to three dimensions of the public discourse that are closely related to the vicissitudes of psychoanalysis. These were: the new policy towards sexuality; the representation of Freud and psychoanalysis in the public press; and clinical directions of psychotherapy in general. Psychoanalysis received the same treatment as sex, which did not exist in the Soviet Union but was widely practised and discussed: it was condemned by the Soviet press and then kept appearing on the pages of newspapers and magazines. Such circulation kept Freud's name alive and present for generations of Soviet citizens and infiltrated everyday speech. The chapter argues this to be an important channel for psychoanalysis to stay in the public consciousness and to keep interest in Freud's ideas alive.

Chapter 3 offers a closer look at the work of Bluma Zeigarnik and her collaboration with Lev Vygotsky and Alexander Luria. It introduces the Soviet period of her career when she developed the theory of thought disturbance, and pathopsychology – a branch of medical psychology concerned with the theory and clinical procedure of diagnosis of mental disturbances. The chapter suggests that Zeigarnik's work shares the theoretical understanding of mental processes and is coherent with Luria and Vygotsky's take on psychoanalysis. A close reading of Zeigarnik's texts and her references to Freud suggests she was properly acquainted with psychoanalytic theory. A parallel reading of Zeigarnik's take on schizophrenia with Freud's work indicates their methodological alignment.

Chapter 4 focuses on the shift in Alexander Luria's career from psychology to physiology, and how his research in neuropsychology and psychophysiology that developed from the 1930s interacted with ideas about the unconscious. It seeks to nuance Luria's transition from psychologist to neuropsychologist and brain researcher, using the archival documents around the defence of his doctorate degree in psychology in Tbilisi and the transfer of it to Moscow in the late 1930s, to argue that the engagement with physiology was both forced and genuine for Luria. The set of archival documents examined in this chapter has not yet been discussed in the existing literature and is most likely presented here for the first time. The chapter outlines some of Luria's ideas on the role of language in the formation of the mind and presents a comparative analysis of his work alongside psychoanalytic concepts.

Chapter 5 turns to the histories of Dmitry Uznadze and Filipp Bassin, two leading voices in Soviet studies on the unconscious. Reading Bassin and Uznadze's main monographs, the chapter suggests that the notion of the 'Soviet unconscious' based on Uznadze's theory of set and established by Bassin as an alternative to Freud was not that much different from Freud's. The critique of Freud that appeared in their work is due to political reasons, and should be read not as a critique, but as a disguise technique that Bassin used to keep the discussion about psychoanalysis alive after 1956. The chapter also presents a review of materials from The International Symposium on the Unconscious, an event held in Tbilisi in 1979 and four Volumes of the symposium papers.

## Part 2: About the method

This book engaged with various sources and historical events:

- general changes in psychology and physiology between 1930 and 1980 as a result of political and ideological pressures;
- biographies and personal connections of 'former' followers of psychoanalysis and theorists engaged with the question of the unconscious: A. Luria, B. Zeigarnik, D. Uznadze, F. Bassin;
- archival materials, mainly from personal files on A. Luria and F. Bassin held in the GARF;
- periodicals, including public newspapers, academic journals and volumes of Soviet Encyclopaedias;
- books dedicated to the discussion of Freud or psychoanalysis 1930–1980;
- materials around particular significant events, such as The Scientific Session Dedicated to the Problem of the Ideological Struggle Against Contemporary Freudism in 1958, including original speeches of its participants, comments and further exchange between participants; as well as the Symposium on the Unconscious in Tbilisi 1979, including four published volumes of materials of this symposium.

In the course of working with these materials, seven key problems emerged that gave shape to how I approach psychoanalysis in this book. I summarize them below.

The first problem is how to understand Freud. Many theorists after Freud discuss his concepts, and we can see how his ideas about the structure of the psyche, the unconscious, the processes of repression and negation, etc. are simultaneously transformed and remain the same. Other concepts such as libido, Oedipus complex, death drive, melancholia are dynamic and are subject to comprehension by theorists outside of psychoanalysis. In fact, Freud left a dictionary of concepts, the general meaning of which thickened within the time and with the help of his careful readers such as Laplanche, Lacan, Klein, Bion.

The consequence of this problem is the production of differences in the reading of Soviet texts, depending on the researcher's understanding of the essence of psychoanalytic concepts.

The second problem is how to understand what psychoanalysis is. Psychoanalysis has already gone beyond clinical institutions and became the basis of the conceptual apparatus of film theory, literary critique, art theory, critical theory, psychosocial studies etc. This book rethinks once again the status of psychoanalysis outside the clinical practice of psychoanalysis, and offers to re-evaluate presented Soviet theories as an extension of psychoanalytic theory in clinical psychology and studies of physiology. However, once transferred to the soil of other disciplines, does psychoanalysis still have a legacy of certain ideas and can we call these studies psychoanalytic, or do they belong to experimental psychology and physiology? Ultimately, could psychoanalysis form interdisciplinary connections?

The book is curious – what if pathopsychology, so widely practiced in the psychiatric system in Soviet and post-Soviet Russia, was in fact a continuation of the application of psychoanalytic ideas? What if Luria's research was still linked to Freudian ideas? What if the theory of set of Uznadze, that constituted the Soviet notion of the unconscious was not different at all from the Freudian or Kleinan unconscious?

The third problem is the modern approach to the consideration of the mind (in many places synonymous with the old-fashioned term *psyche*). For example, today the ideas of psycho-physiological unity sound completely different to us than to Soviet psychologists and physiologists. The terminological apparatus of Soviet psychologists is full of terms from biology, physiology, and neuropsychology. However, today there is not only a time gap, but also a methodological one between these terms and terms in contemporary neuroscience.

Luria, for example, at some point calls psychoanalysis a monistic psychology that understands the work of the mind in its unity. He studies brain damage but his writing is interested in the linguistic effects of it. He writes on aphasia, but his focus is on the disorganization of semantic fields, rather than on links between brain lesion and disturbance. Uznadze's notion of the 'set' (*ustanovka*) assumes a combination of psychological and physiological factors in psychic reactions. Nevertheless, while operating on the level of physiological terminology, these studies do not exclude consideration of the individual as a complex psychological constellation. They also do not equate nervous and brain mechanisms with the mechanisms of the psyche. That's why Soviet studies of brain and terminology for the contemporary researcher can sound misleading, if taken without consideration of how psycho-physiological unity was assumed in the systemic approach of Soviet scientists.

The fourth problem concerns historiography. Revisiting the chosen historical era for this book serves two purposes: refining our understanding of history in light of new findings and reinterpreting already known facts in a different way. There is a growing body of research on the unique characteristics of Soviet science as a whole, but this has not yet been applied to the history of psychoanalysis. At the same time, our understanding of psychoanalysis has expanded beyond its clinical applications, offering new insights into its potential relevance in different contexts. Little work has been done to explore how this broader understanding could shed light on the meaning of Soviet psychologists' texts within their societal and scientific framework at the time.

The fifth problem is political. Since psychoanalysis in Soviet times developed in the context of communism, Soviet ideas were criticized indiscriminately, along with the entire political system and its science as a whole. The solution to this problem is to recognize the original status of Soviet science and consider the relevance and possibility of applying the ideas of Soviet psychologists outside the communist political system. In other words, it is necessary to separate the opposition to 'communist' ideas from the theoretical ideas of Soviet psychologists. Proctor is trying to make a similar move, reflecting on the significance of the ideas of Luria and Vygotsky for the revolutionary movement today (2016, p. 157).

The question of who a subject of psychoanalysis is also a political one. For example, Vyrgioti highlights how psychoanalytic theory is a colonial theory and at the same time has a potential solution to deconstruct colonial discourse, as Freud

> draws on cannibalism as a colonial representation of racial difference to argue that social life depends on the repression of cannibalistic wishes. On the other hand, in modelling the process of identification upon cannibalistic wishes, Freud challenges the dichotomy between the hegemonic, white civilised subject and the racialised, cannibalistic other.
>
> (Vyrgioti, 2022, p. 79)

Also, psychoanalysis is designed to work with the white Western individual and originates in capitalist values. How does it work then for a communist society? When thinking about the individual in Soviet psychology, who was desexualized and deprived of a private life, a question arises: could they be a subject of psychoanalysis? When the core notion of sexuality had to be censored from the discussion, will it still be a psychoanalytic discussion?

The sixth, important, problem, is how to understand and to define 'Soviet' and therefore how to approach it. While the Soviet Union was a huge country that united different cultures, languages and nationalities, it is a great generalization to use the term 'Soviet' to refer to it as a unified entity. Geographically, the academic activity covered by the current research happened predominantly in Moscow, Saint Petersburg and Tbilisi. The geography of origin of Soviet psychologists that are subjects of my research is more varied: Lithuania, Belarus, Ukraine, Tatarstan and Georgia. Nationality is Jewish and Georgian. That brings us to perhaps suggest that psychoanalysis could have been a mode of thinking generated by outsiders, and thus the notion of 'Soviet' is not exactly applicable to them as it homogenizes a rather diverse cohort.

Still, when we think about science, standards of Soviet psychology and Soviet physiology originated in the political context of 1930s. It was shaped by purges and anti-bourgeois campaigns. It was also shaped later by the Pavlov Session and had features of what is called Stalinist science, so there were some shared Soviet features despite the individual specifics of scientists.

Approaches to the mind in psychology and physiology were unified and standardized, and as was already noted in this book, the centralization of science meant that findings from Moscow were delivered to Russified regions.

The scientific community was also in tune with the global scientific society to some extent, as it was not fully isolated behind the Iron Curtain as was previously thought. Also, Luria, Zeigarnik, Bassin and Uznadze knew at least one foreign language and most of them studied abroad and were well-connected with international colleagues and up-to date with publications in their subjects. From the late 1950s all of them travelled abroad (apart from Uznadze, who was dead by that time) to participate in conferences, so their exchanges could have been even more free. Thus, even though the synonyms of Soviet can sometimes be 'backwards' and 'totalitarian' or 'isolated' this is not exactly true and represents a reductionist view of Soviet ideas. However, the science was shaped by the Soviet state, and it would also be a mistake not to consider this.

The seventh problem is the atrocities of Soviet psychiatry and the collaboration with the regime to persecute dissidents. While writing about psy-disciplines in Soviet Union it is difficult not to slip into all or nothing narrative, and this book might not be able to avoid it. The psychiatric system of Soviet Union was punitive in many ways since 1936 and yet a lot of valuable insights, for example from Zeigarnik work with schizophrenia, can be taken from it. I will address peculiarities of the relationships with the State when writing about Luria, Zeigarnik, Bassin and Uznadze, who worked in the psychiatric institutions or related to them organizations.

These will each be addressed in their complexities further.

### A note on archives

> If I distrust my memory – neurotics, as we know, do so to a remarkable extent, but normal people have every reason for doing so as well – I am able to supplement and guarantee its working by making a note in writing.... I have only to bear in mind the place where this 'memory' has been deposited and I can then 'reproduce' it at any time I like, with the certainty that it will have remained unaltered and so have escaped the possible distortions to which it might have been subjected in my actual memory.
>
> (Freud, 1925, p. 227)

It is a widely held view that when dealing with history, researchers should base their studies on historical facts. But what if facts are not that factual, and what if the work of fantasy, as in psychic reality, impact the memory giving facts a different meaning? How do we uncover distortions? In psychoanalysis, the speech of the subject is used as evidence. Like a policeman in an American movie, who warns the criminal about the right to keep silent, as 'everything you say might be used in the court', a psychoanalyst uses what is said to recreate the reality of the patient. A psychoanalyst also acts even more brutally, using the silence 'against' the subject as well. What is said and what is silenced, thus, becomes the material for analytic interpretation. As a psychosocial researcher who explores history, I employ this way of treating what was said and what was silenced in texts that I was studying.

While a memory of the ordinary subject is full of gaps, transformations, and distortions, as is seen by examples in psychoanalysis, the archival collection, on the other hand, appears as a store where the evidence is preserved 'as it is'. But we should not be naïve and assume that archives store 'everything'. One should consider gaps and distortions made by the authorities, restrictions of access, and the reasons why some materials are selected to be open for the public. The Soviet authorities decided what to keep and what to destroy, and this is the first layer of memory distortion. By selecting specific archival material from the whole range and leaving others aside, researchers organized the second layer of memory distortion. The third layer of memory distortion is of a psychological nature. As Figes (2008) shows in his research on people who survived the purges of the early Stalinist years, many of them did not share their origin (aristocratic background, for example) and their true beliefs even with their spouses and children. The period introduced in the title locates the beginning of this story in 1930; however, the research was actually commenced between 2019 and 2023, and was influenced by the knowledge I have as a researcher. Knowledge of psychoanalysis, which I studied for many years, knowledge of psychology as I was educated in post-Soviet university that still followed more or less the same standards for education, knowledge of unspoken kind, because I was born in Soviet Union and raised by two generations of people who was formed as Soviets.

Speaking about the collection of knowledge and discursive formations in society, Foucault sees the archive in the broader sense as the combination of sources of gained knowledge. But he dedicates to archives not just a storage function: "The archive is first the law of what can be said, the system that governs the appearance of statements as unique events" (Foucault, 1972, p. 129). The method to research that archival field – *archaeology* – is not "the search for the beginning" for Foucault:

> It designates the general theme of a description that questions the already-said at the level of its existence: of the enunciative function that operates within it, of the discursive formation, and the general archive system to which it belongs. Archaeology describes discourses as practices specified in the element of the archive.
>
> (p. 131)

This book presupposes that the whole field of knowledge about psychoanalysis in Soviet times is an archive, including not only archival documents, but also original writings around psychoanalysis in Soviet times and existing studies of the history of that time. Applied to the archival field of knowledge on psychoanalysis in the Soviet Union, we see those distortions in operation. First, we have pre-established histories or already made studies and series of names, events and texts already assigned to psychoanalysis by researchers. Second, we have evidence of changes in state approaches to psychoanalysis throughout the timeline 1900s-1920s-1930s-1950s-1970s-1980s, when it was 'allowed' and 'prohibited' by the Party ideology, revealed by archival documents collected and preserved by the State. Third, we have names that were never mentioned or assigned to psychoanalysis in the Soviet Union, i.e., were excluded from the discursive formation.

To break with what was drawn on by previous research as belonging to that history, I've also included newspapers and academic periodicals, as well as the constellation of monographs and books, which I treat as primary sources and analyse as archival documents. I paid attention to new and recurrent names, editors, publishing houses and numbers of copies of books (*terazh*). I've included styles of writings, styles of criticism, references and the absence of references as important parts of this archive. Through simultaneous analysis of multiple archival parts, I aimed to find and to recognize their inherent discursive formation(s) and to widen the territory of this 'archive'. To my surprise, this approach proved to be rather fruitful. It explained certain gaps and inconsistencies, as well as offered new interpretations of already familiar events and existing materials. I found myself engaging in not only psychosocial research but the work of the historian: chasing lost causes, finding clues in footnotes, piecing a story together from fragmentary evidence, I had to collect information literally bit by bit, following footnotes and brief mentions, sometimes finding important information in completely unrelated sources.

To a certain extent, I've included my memory in this archive too. The memory of my grandmother's books who, every summer from when I was seven through to my late teenage years, ensured that, alongside the classic literature, I read the Soviet authors she selected for me: books about Soviet youth and then more problematic books of Soviet dissidents. The memory of my grandfather's jokes, who was a teenager during World War II and told me stories of his youth after the war times. Some of his jokes I only understood while reading Waterlow's book on Stalinist jokes which I'll discuss further. The memory of my parents' youth stories, their times at university and summers of building railways deep in the country East, sounded to me alike stories I read in books. The memory of what I've studied as a medical student in Belarus and a clinical psychologist student in Russia.

### *Evidential (conjectural) paradigm*

This extended notion of the archive had an impact on the set of methods chosen for my research. It shifted the focus from the search for major discoveries to the importance of small details.

Carlo Ginzburg formulated this approach through the notion of the 'evidential (or conjectural) paradigm' (1989, p. 96). This method unites Morelli – an art critic known for recognizing painting forgery, Freud – known for recognizing the unconscious in slips of the tongue, and Conan Doyle – the creator of the fictional detective Sherlock Holmes. "In each case, infinitesimal traces permit the comprehension of a deeper, otherwise unattainable reality: traces – more precisely, symptoms (in the case of Freud), clues (in the case of Sherlock Holmes), pictorial marks (in the case of Morelli" (Ginzburg, 1989, p. 101).

An example of this method is a psychoanalytic approach to the analysis of data. It can be formulated through several principles, such as reading between the lines, attention to minor details, attention to inconsistencies and contradictions, attention to negation. All of them can be found in various of Freud's texts. In *The Interpretation of Dreams* (1900), Freud discusses mechanisms of the dream by explaining the work of censorship. Most important for him were minor details, in which unconscious ideas lurk and stay unnoticed, unless we highlight their presence by special effort. And what is more, when a person recounts the dream, the work of censorship continues to minimize the importance of these details in speech, for example through additions like 'it is not significant', 'the minor detail there', 'small piece', etc.

When interpreting a dream, Freud asked a patient to tell the dream twice, and made notes about places in the narrative which were not the same during the second round. Freud linked this to the logic of censorship, arguing that in order to avoid emotional encounters with sensitive bits of the dream, a patient would distort these 'grey' parts when speaking. With negation in speech the aim is the same, to establish distance from emotionally charged material.

Altogether, this approach constitutes reading between lines, based on the presupposition that what is spoken is not what is meant. In other words, for Freud the work of censorship is constantly present in speech and in order to find truth we need to assume another meaning of what was said. I apply the same logic when reading the texts in this book, because they derive from the period of explicit censorship in science and in society in general. However, this does not mean I treat every text as having this critical distortion; rather, I allow for its possible presence and see what kind of new interpretations this assumption brings.

From the close reading of texts, for example, I began to realize that the appearance of Freud's name in Zeigarnik's writings is consistent throughout 1935–1980. Although in some texts it is only mentioned once, in others Freud's ideas are discussed at length –she is also known to have been reading lectures on Freud and Freudians from 1956. In contrast, in Luria's texts Freud's name disappeared after the mid-1930s. Bassin engaged with Freud's ideas in 1930, shifted to physiology during the period 1935–1956, and until the late 1980s was consistently critical of psychoanalysis, publishing around five articles a year dedicated to the 'critique' of psychoanalysis and demonstrating a very thorough knowledge of it. Uznadze's engagement with Freud is also interrupted at some point. It is difficult to trace when exactly the change occurred in Uznadze's texts, as his main monograph was only published in Russian in 1966. If we do not interpret these changes critically, the conclusion will simply reiterate already existing narrative – psychoanalysis was 'banned' in Soviet Russia in the 1930s and psychologists were critical of it. If we allow the presence of the critical distortion, it is interesting to see how Bassin was becoming Freud's critic after Khrushchev's 'secret speech' and the beginning of the de-Stalinization campaign. In the same vein we can see Zeigarnik's lectures, that she began to read around the same time. For Luria, who was regularly persecuted and questioned for 15 years (between 1924 and 1939) for being Freudian, perhaps not to speak about Freud was not of much theoretical concern.

## The socio-historical dimension

This book follows the approach of revisionist histories from the late 20th century, which highlight often-overlooked historical figures who navigated and survived under authoritarian and repressive conditions (e.g., Fitzpatrick, Yasnitsky, Kouzulin). While paying close attention to specific details, I also aim to consider the broader context in which the events and ideas discussed in this book emerged.

Recent studies on Soviet history have explored various aspects of life and science in the Soviet Union, revealing the complex socio-historical environment of the time. This book include research on pedology (Byford, 2020), humour (Waterlow, 2018), social structures (Yurchak, 2005), and informal networks (Ledeneva, 1998). Additionally, broader studies on Soviet psychology and the 'Stalinist tradition' (Yasnitsky, 2019; Kozulin, 1984) as well as Stalinist science (Krementsov, 1996; Pollock, 2006) have demonstrated that nothing in Soviet Russia was immune to political influence.

This understanding shaped my approach and informed the structure of my investigation, which introduces practices from the Soviet period used to navigate life under the regime, as discussed in the next chapter. These practices help us understand how psychoanalysis continued to be discussed, disseminated, and adapted over time, in response to the shifting political and social landscape.

## Shifting the binary discourse

In this book, I intend to shift from the binary discourse that Yurchak catches in his work, observing the phrase 'the Soviet regime',

> with the myriad assumptions often packed into it – and in the use of binary categories to describe Soviet reality such as oppression and resistance, repression and freedom, the state and the people, official economy and second economy, official culture and counterculture, totalitarian

language and counterlanguage, public self and private self, truth and lie, reality and dissimulation, morality and corruption, and so on.

(Yurchak, 2005, p. 5)

Contrary to such reductive approaches (Yurchak, 2005, p. 9) he suggests reconstructing Soviet life in its complexity. Following Yurchak, instead of claiming that psychoanalysis was present or absent during the period 1930–1980, I show how practices consonant with psychoanalysis emerged out of early collaborations with psychoanalytic theory, how psychoanalytic ideas continued to be explored within other disciplines such as psychology and physiology, and how this was organized to be possible.

Yurchak (2005, p. 14) further examines 'authoritative discourse', a term he borrows from Bakhtin, in order to show how the reality 'fixed' by this discourse started to produce new meanings without opposing it. Authoritative discourse has two main features: 1) it has a special 'script' in which it is coded and sharply demarcated from other types of discourse; being not dependent upon them, it precedes them and cannot be changed by them, and 2) other discourses "having to refer to it, quote it, praise it, interpret it, apply it, and so forth, but they cannot, for example, interfere with its code and change it" (Yurchak, 2005, p. 15 quoting from Bakhtin 1994, 342–343). We see the establishment of this discourse as early as the mid-1920s when psychoanalysis became 'bourgeois, idealist' theory as opposed to the Marxist-Leninist view of the mind, that by the 1950s was codified as a form of Pavlovian theory. In the 1930s it was already impossible to argue the social nature of mental disturbance and biological explanations took the dominant place, although they did not yet consolidate around a specific theory. By the 1950s, the discourse centred on the name of Pavlov and reflex theory. And even after 1962 when more scientists were allowed by authorities, they all had to be 'domestic' (*otechestvennyie*). This 'script' and multiple references to it were apparent in the public press, perhaps not surprisingly, as state newspapers and journals were increasingly censored. However, as we will see in the next chapter, from the discussion around Freud in academic production, *Pravda* and other newspapers, some knowledge about Freud slipped into these pages too.

Despite the fact that "during the late Soviet period, the form of ideological representations – documents, speeches, ritualized practices, slogans, posters, monuments, and urban visual propaganda – became increasingly normalized, ubiquitous, and predictable" (Yurchak, 2005, p. 14), Yurchak found that citizens were able to overcome the authoritative discourse without just opposing it. "In most contexts these unanimous acts, gestures, and utterances of support did not refer to the literal meaning of ideological statements, resolutions, and figures, but rather performed a different role" (Yurchak, 2005, p. 16). The language of newspapers, speeches of the party leaders and local authorities were standardized and unified. And if ordinary citizens used the structure to perform different dimensions of life, why not assume that in discussion around Freud and psychoanalysis similar practices could be found too? After all, these were the same citizens who lived everyday life and had to adjust to the authoritative discourse.

To understand how exactly it was possible, Yurchak suggests we need to follow Derrida:

> The conventionality of a speech act implies that it must be formulated according to a recognized 'coded' or 'iterable' model – that is, it must function as a citation that is repeatable in an endless number of contexts (Derrida 1977, 191–92). However, the exhaustive knowledge of context cannot be achieved because any context is open to broader description and because contexts in which new citations of the same speech act can appear are potentially infinite (Derrida 1977, 185–86).
> 
> (quoted from Yurchack, 2005, p. 20)

To put it simply, the reiterations of Pavlov's name as found in the publications of that time do not necessarily refer to Pavlovian ideas, and most likely refer to the presence of the authoritative discourse. This is something that yet awaits to be studied in more detail: to what extent did Soviet psychologists truly follow the ideas of Pavlov? If we apply this idea to the criticism of Freud, we can also say that phrases like 'bourgeois, idealist Freud' or 'Freud was too inclined to biological explanations' are phrases that refer to the authoritative discourse, rather than indicating the position of the author.

The explicit and unspoken rules of this era have been sufficiently studied (Kozulin, 1984; Krementsov, 1996; Ledeneva, 1998; Yurchak, 2005; Waterlow, 2018; Yasnitsky, 2019), which allows us to summarize several of its main features. First, in thinking about what was said by someone we need to allow multiple meanings of it, depending on the context and circumstances. Second, the language of ideology is used to move within the structure of society. At the same time, 'a speaker' of this language could absolutely disagree with his own statement. If we apply these features to the studied topic, we lose certainty that the public statements of psychologists represented their real position, and the criticism of Freud in their work expresses their real attitude towards psychoanalysis.

Overall, Yurchak illustrates how

> the performative shift of authoritative discourse that occurred in the 1950s and 1960s allowed Soviet people to develop a complexly differentiating relationship to ideological meanings, norms, and values. Depending on the context, they might reject a certain meaning, norm, or value, be apathetic about another, continue actively subscribing to a third, creatively reinterpret a fourth, and so on.
> 
> (Yurchak, 2005, pp. 28–29)

"In other words", he continues, "the performative dimension of authoritative discourse started to play a much greater role than its constative dimension" (Yurchak, 2005, p. 37). This is exactly the period when the Freud Session in 1958 took place and the discussion was opened around the issue of 'Soviet studies on the unconscious'. The performative dimension of this session will be discussed further. However, the inclusion of both performative and authoritative dimensions of the discourse brought into consideration the question of mechanism, of what could support that division. This is how the notion of splitting became an integral part of this book's study.

## *Splitting*

Splitting in psychology is a mechanism that allows a person to live through difficult experiences and emotions by separating them into 'good' and 'bad', idealized or devalued categories. Splitting as a mechanism of disconnection is found in language, public behaviour and styles of criticism, and has been outlined by Krementsov (1996) as a main characteristic of Stalinist science. That splitting created oppositions such as 'Russian' and 'Western' science, loyal and disloyal to the Party, communist and bourgeoise, etc. Yet despite how paradoxical it might sound, the work of splitting in Soviet society also brought the possibility of integration.

Krementsov (1996) and Pollock (2006) pointed to this kind of splitting and showed that reference to the statements of Lenin, Stalin, Marx and Engels was an obligatory part of the introduction to scientific work and the structure of science under Stalin and did not necessarily indicate genuine engagement with their ideas. Waterlow's work on humour in Stalinist times investigated the splitting produced by jokes and anecdotes as a form of resistance to official ideology and a way to sustain identifications. There he introduced the idea of the crosshatching – an "unconscious mixing of official and unofficial discourses, values and assumptions" (Waterlow, 2018, p. 6). Ledeneva (1998) captures what I call splitting in the practice of *blat* – an alternative socio-economic form of the device,[4] which was simultaneously denied and performed by the participants of her study. The emergence of informal practices, including *blat*, organized the overall splitting of the economy in Brezhnev's times and emergence of the second economy and black markets. In academia, as Kozulin (1984) showed, criticism as a form of expression was widely used in the field of psychology to bring to the reader ideas that were 'prohibited' by official discourse. This is the incomplete list of examples of the encounter with the work of splitting in studies around Soviet era. But this incompleteness points exactly outside of the binary, and this is something that revisionists in social history, like Krylova (2000) objected to in Kotkin's view on strategies available under totalitarian rule, because life strategies under ideological pressure were much more varied than just 'speaking Bolshevik' or being a dissident. She problematizes the so-called Stalinist subject, who was allowed two positions: "a complete inner break with Stalinist reality or a complete identification with it" (Krylova, 2000, p. 145) and suggests another resolution: "the Stalinist man, who will be allowed to internalise official ideology without being able to identify with it" (Krylova, 2000, p. 145). The central question for her is how officially propagated ideas work in people's lives, and what were the consequences if they were internalized and practiced (Krylova, 2000, p. 146). For me an important point here is allowance of the co-existence of the official discourse and alternative discourses that I think were not only practiced on the level of individual lives, but through certain individuals allowed psychoanalysis to continue to influence ideas while being officially prohibited.

The work of splitting occupies a central place in my analysis of the chosen period. With repressions and purges, the splits between private and public life could, at times, become dramatic. What was said in public often aimed to address the authorities rather than convey an authentic message. In such circumstances, reading beyond what was officially produced is only possible if this act of splitting is consistently kept in mind. I consider it a defining characteristic of the era, inherently present in any act of enunciation. This perspective guides my efforts to reconstruct new meanings when researching articles, monographs, and public speeches by Soviet psychologists who, at some point in their scientific careers, engaged with the study of psychoanalytic theory.

## Notes

1 Although in English this notion appears as Freudianism, the correct Soviet version is Freudism. This term echoes Marxism, Leninism and all other -isms appeared in the Soviet Union after the Revolution of 1917.
2 Both terms refer to the importance of the unconscious reaction of the patient to the illness and unconscious relations to the doctor as factors of recovery.
3 See the article of Alexandra Brokman (2018a): "The possibility of influencing human organism through words, and to an extent also through other stimuli, lay at the heart of Soviet approaches to psychotherapy".
4 In Russia, *blat* is a colloquial term to denote ways of getting things done through personal contacts, associated with using connections, pulling strings and exchanging favours. In the Soviet Union *blat* contacts were commonly used to obtain goods and services in short supply or to circumvent formal procedures (Global Informality Project).

Chapter 1

# Histories of psychoanalysis in Soviet Russia and its discontents

Victor Ovcharenko, one of the most prolific encyclopaedists of psychoanalysis in the Russian speaking field, suggests the following periods in the history of Russian psychoanalysis can be identified (Ovcharenko, 1999, pp. 341–353):

1 The educational 1904–1910
   The period when Freud's works appeared and spread in the professional networks. Psychoanalysis is supported not only by psychiatrists, but also psychoanalytic ideas were popular with artists and writers.
2 The adaptive 1910–1914
   The period in which links were established with European psychoanalysts and institutions. The rise of working groups in Russia, and publications of Russian psychoanalysts in the European journals.
3 The disintegrative 1914–1922
   The period of the reduction of activity due to the First World War and the Civil War.
4 The institutional 1922–1932
   The period of an attempt to institutionalize psychoanalysis. Wide publishing and research activity.
5 The latent 1932–1956
   The period usually seen as the termination of psychoanalysis. Ovcharenko argues the lack of evidence for the presence of psychoanalysis does not prove its absence.
6 The bilateral 1956–1989
   In this period psychoanalysis was still criticized and Freud's works did not openly appear in publications, however, a number of researchers engaged with psychoanalytic ideas in their publications and were a source of knowledge on psychoanalysis for the public.
7 The integrative 1989–to date (written in 1999)
   The period is characterized by the re-emergence of activity around and rehabilitation of psychoanalysis. In this period, we see the re-publication of Freud's works, the establishment of psychoanalytic associations, societies, and institutes, as well as new books and journals.

Within this periodization, Ovcharenko, with the passion of a collector, created a list of Soviet psychologists and psychiatrists who practiced psychoanalysis or were somehow involved in activities connected with it. His 432-page volume titled *Russian Psychoanalysts* [*Russkie Psikhoanalitiki*] (2000) contains information on names, organizations, journals, book series and a near-complete psychoanalytic bibliography of the Soviet period. He offers brief histories of 200 people engaged with psychoanalysis in different times of their careers. Despite the impressive number of people listed in there, a reader does not get much detailed information about how exactly some of the names were engaged in psychoanalysis or about their theories. We still don't know much about how and why these people were engaged with psychoanalytic ideas.

Similar situation is found in Soviet psychology, which is still considered an under-researched area. Contemporary historian of Soviet psychology, Sergei Bogdanchikov (2009), criticizes Russian historians of psychology for unclear formulations, the absence of a coherent picture of the time period, and a lack of study around the theories themselves.

Especially in the period 1932–1956, when psychology was endangered as a discipline, although theorists of psychology still existed there were no faculties for students to study in. Bogdanchikov (2018) calls this the situation of 'generals without soldiers', meaning that there were still people who could teach, but there were no institutions in which they could teach and no students to undertake their studies. In a way, Bogdanchikov brings to our attention a very important question: how can we study the history of a discipline that lost its institutions for so many years?

The complication was not only in the fact that psychological laboratories were closed, and former psychologists sought new areas for their professional development. In the years between 1930 and 1950, Soviet psychologists developed their ideas under high ideological pressure and in the harsh conditions of The Great Patriotic War. The comparatively free period from 1950 to 1980 still bore witness to the great impact of strict ideologies and the persecution of dissidents. These ideological shifts changed the language of scholars, many of whom won't have known a period in which they could write freely, whilst those who were older had been operating under repressive conditions for several decades. Authors were required to consider many factors, including reference to Party leaders, a necessary attribute of writing at that time. Western citations were either limited or prohibited entirely. A scholar could only engage with ideologically 'permitted' sources. The censorship system was strict, and the consequences of writing outside of this system could be life-threatening (Krementsov, 1996; Pollock, 2006, Yasnitsky, 2019). How can we study the history of a discipline that not only lost its institutions, but also lost its vocabulary to ideology?

Naturally, these complications puzzled many Russian historians who were writing about Soviet psychology. Those who wrote from within Soviet times also brought into their research distortions they were not critical of due to their position 'within' the system. An example of this could be the case of the Vygotsky 'ban'. Well-known historians of psychology in Soviet times, like Petrovsky and Zhdan, always highlighted the fact that Vygotsky's writings were banned and disappeared from references for a period between 1930 and 1960. A new generation of scholars, however, challenged these assertions. For example, Yasnitsky (2015, pp. 128–153) concluded that the claim that there was a 'ban' was more a tradition of thinking but, in reality, there is no compelling evidence to support this. Historians just inherited the views of the previous scholars, and no one really doubted the established narrative. Similarly, in the study correlating participation with and connections between Soviet psychologists and Western colleagues, Yasnitsky shows that Russian works were published in English and German sometimes before they appeared in Russian, and that references to Western articles were present in some Soviet writings before they were officially published (Yasnitsky, 2012a, pp. 110–112). This goes against the 'Iron curtain' narrative, that was for a long time present in the history of Soviet psychology. Being revisionists when it comes to breaking traditional narratives of the history of Soviet psychology, neither Yasnitsky nor Bogdanchikov dedicate space to the relationship between Soviet psychologists and psychoanalysis in their work. This is interesting, considering the huge interest in and awareness of Freud's work, not only amongst doctors but also high-ranking politicians and intellectuals of the time. And thanks to Ovcharenko we have a detailed list of them. It looks like historians more happily acknowledge the influence of, say, Gestalt psychology, and uncritically the roots of Soviet psychology are normally linked to Sechenov or Pavlov, meaning that somehow there is a resistance against including psychoanalysis in the scope.

The situation, however, might not be specific to Russia, as Yakushko writes regarding US psychology: "Direct influences of psychoanalytic theories on key psychology figures such as Erickson, Piaget, Vygotsky, Luria, Frankl, and many others who were openly affiliated with psychoanalysis, are typically omitted or minimized in psychology textbooks" (2021, p. 639).

My research suggests that, more broadly, the problem with studies of psychoanalysis or psychology in Soviet times is of a discursive kind. Scholars of psychoanalysis (and of Soviet psychology) attempted to reconstruct the *development* of the discipline, while I think we are dealing with the history of *survival*. If we agree to ignore linear development and try to make sense of what was happening in the field and with people, both on the level of events and ideas, there is a potential for more understanding. This chapter attempts to implement such an approach.

## An analysis of the Soviet and its discontents

The following paragraphs will present a summary of the history of psychoanalysis in Soviet Russia in its current formulation.

Between 1900 and 1920, Freud's books were widely translated and published in Russian, even though psychoanalytic texts were accessible for Russian doctors without translations, as most of them spoke at least German and English and regularly travelled to Europe for study and exchange. Freud's *Interpretation of Dreams* was translated into Russian before it was translated into any other language (Miller, 1998, p. xi). During the second decade of the 20$^{th}$ century there were 22 more translations. Between 1922 and 1928, the Psychological and Psychoanalytic Library [*Psikhologicheskaia i Psikhoanaliticheskaia Biblioteka*] in the state publishing house [*Gosizdatelstvo*] also published a series of translations of Carl Jung, Karl Abraham, Ernest Jones, Victor Tausk, Sandor Ferenczi, Melanie Klein and other psychoanalysts.

Both Lou-Andreas Salome and Sabina Spielrein, the only women allowed at Freud's Wednesday meetings, were born in the Russian Empire. Psychoanalytic theory informed many early Soviet psychiatrists' and psychologists' practices and stimulated their future theoretical development, such as Ivan Ermakov, Otto and Vera Schmidt, Sabina Spielrein, Nikolay Osipov, Tatiana Rosental, Nikolay Vyrubov, Yuri Kannabikh, Mikheil Asatiani, and Alexander Bernstein. Vibrant centres for psychoanalysis before it moved to Moscow were in Odesa, Kharkiv, Kyiv, at that time part of the Russian Empire, nowadays Ukraine (Pushrakeva and Romanov, 2000). Pushrakeva and Romanov (2000) points to the fact that Freud's reference to psychoanalysis in Russia (Freud, 1914) was linked to activity in Odesa, where Moshe Wulff, who later headed the Russian Psychoanalytic Society, worked. Filipp Bassin, an important figure for Soviet discussion around psychoanalysis between 1950s and 1980s, first encountered psychoanalysis in Kharkiv, where he studied and worked before moving to Moscow.

Many intellectuals in Soviet Russia were fascinated by psychoanalysis. Among them were the famous director Sergei Eisenstein, writer Andrey Bely, thinker Vasily Rozanov, and philosopher Mikhail Bakhtin (Etkind, 1997, pp. 5, 41, 179). The politician Leon Trotsky supported psychoanalysis and tried to combine ideas from Freud and Pavlov (Etkind, 1997, p. 229; Roudinesco, 1990, p. 38). Before moving to the Soviet Union, the State economist Eugen Varga was a member of the Hungarian Psychoanalytic Society and often visited Freud's house for weekly Wednesday meetings. In 1921, Varga worked with Lenin, before becoming Stalin's economic adviser in the 1930s. Between 1920 and 1925, he participated in the activities of the Russian Psychoanalytic Society, even taking up the role of vice-president (Tögel, 2006). The engagement of politicians and the support from the State promised a great future for those in the field of psychoanalysis when the first ever state-supported Psychoanalytic Institute opened in Soviet Russia in 1922 (Miller, 1998, p. xi). Citing

Lenin, Etkind represents psychoanalysis after the Revolution as a fashion: "Freud's theory is a kind of popular fad, nowadays" (Miller, 1998, p. 179).

Among those enthusiasts was a young psychologist Alexander Luria, who moved to Moscow in 1923 and immediately engaged with the Psychoanalytic Institute where he became the secretary. Being already involved in organising the Psychoanalytic Society in Kazan, which had received a warm welcome from Freud, Luria continued his activity in Moscow and between 1920 and 1930 regularly submitted minutes of meetings of the psychoanalytic society into the Bulletin of the International Psychoanalytic Society and papers to the *Internationale Zeitschrift für Psychoanalyse*.

However, political changes including the rise of Stalin created circumstances for the ideological suppression of psychoanalysis. With Trotsky's decline in popularity in the Party and general transformations in Soviet psychology in the mid-1920s, the enthusiasm for psychoanalysis waned. Soviet newspapers provide plenty of evidence that public attacks on psychoanalysis had started as early as 1924. The State Psychoanalytic Institute was closed in 1925. Two years later, in 1927, Luria resigned as secretary of the Psychoanalytic Society, the same year as its collapse and Trotsky's defeat (Etkind, 1997). Parting with psychoanalytic ideas was not immediate; in 1930–1931 Luria and Vygotsky were still noted for their 'ideological mistakes' and 'lack of vigilance' towards psychoanalysis and Freudism (Leibin, 1991). There is a record in Vygotsky's Notebook of a conference meeting in 1933 which he attended, with participation of Vera Schmidt, V.A. Averbukh, M.S. Pevzner in which Schmidt presented thesis on the development of the psychoneurosis of the child, with multiple references to Freud and ideas around the unconscious, drives, etc. (Zavershneva and van der Veer, 2017, p. 451). After the decree of VKP (b) by the Central Committee 'On Pedological Perversions in the Narkompros System' in 1936,[1] diversity in psychology was officially banned and the purges of 1937–8 left no space for an open discussion of psychoanalysis. From then on, published works by Soviet psychologists only referenced Freud in a critical manner or excluded him completely, as well as many other Western authors.

Certainly, as Etkind formulates it, Russia was 'captured' by psychoanalysis in the years leading up to its 'ban'. The engagement of high-ranking politicians and the support of the State promised a great future in the field of psychoanalysis. However, like the promised great future for all new Soviet citizens, it never happened. Freud returned only after the fall of the Soviet Union and establishment of the new country – the Russian Federation. However, this return of Freud was different. One may say all sorts and variations of psychotherapeutic theories and approaches floated throughout Russia whilst Freud was represented as outdated. As one of the witnesses of the second arrival of psychoanalysis remembers,

> Of course there is no doubt that Sigmund Freud is an authority, but he was always regarded as a rather elderly and patriarchal background

figure who had written something wise and evidently true but so long ago as to be probably inapplicable to us. I think that this idea was not so much a Russian idea as something we picked up by reading Western sources.

(Cote, 1998. p. 104)

And if the notion of 'outdated Freud' was picked up from the Western sources, what was Russia's original idea of Freud? Alex Kozulin (1984), Alexander Etkind (1997), Martin A. Miller (1998), Elisabeth Roudinesco (1990), Alberto Angelini (1988, 2008) and Dmitry Rozhdestvenskii (2009)[2] have some answers to that question. To summarize their position, possible reasons for its dissolution and ban in the 1930s were pre- revolutionary Russian and Soviet features of psychoanalysis, such as: the political effects born of a combination of Marxism and psychoanalysis; the lack of clinical development. Both resulted into gradual dissolution of engagement with psychoanalytic theory.

I suggest, however, that the disappearance of psychoanalysis from the official scientific discussions was concerned with Russification of the Soviet Science, the need to eradicate any bourgeoise traces from it and suffered indirectly complications from growing antisemitic tendencies. It was a result of greater changes in science, that prompted splitting into publicly accepted and hidden developments in it.

## *The political effects born of a combination of Marxism and psychoanalysis*

Roudinesco, Miller, and Etkind argued that psychoanalysis meant a lot for early Soviet Russia because of its possible compatibility with Marxist ideologies, so the plan of politicians who were engaged with psychoanalysis was to use it for the good of the new country. Of course, there is nothing specific in such a bond, as the whole of science in the Soviet Union, as we will see later, was highly politicized at those times.

Loren Graham (1967) shows how Soviet science was adopted by the state in Soviet Russia, and how it worked to serve its needs. The invention of the new State after the October Revolution of 1917 brought crucial changes into all structures of the formal state, including science and academia. However, the sciences benefited from this bond with the State. This argument is also developed by Krementsov (1996), so it is difficult to conclude that psychoanalysis in particular was highly charged, politically, or that it was a specific issue in relation to psychoanalysis.

On one hand, perhaps, it is better to say that psychoanalysis had to engage with politics in order to survive, as was the demand of the Soviet State. However, even though many authors tried to engage with psychoanalysis and Marxism, the main psychoanalytic theoreticians – among them, Ivan Ermakov, Sabina Spielrein, Vera and Otto Schmidt, Nikolay Osipov, and others – stayed out of political engagement. Attempts by Luria and Vygotsky to comment on psychoanalysis and Marxism in their work on the death drive were seen as rather naïve, and perhaps made under the influence of the general tendency (Proctor, 2020). Nevertheless, Kozulin notices that translators and scholars who were researching the works of Lev Vygotsky found that English texts cut a lot of references to Marx, considering them an ideological gesture. Vygotsky, on the other hand, was genuinely interested in Marxism and his references are thoughtful (Kozulin, 1984; Etkind, 1997, p. 230). Only after that discovery were correct translations made. On the other hand, since Trotsky supported psychoanalysis, it might have influenced others in the party or created an air of mystery for psychoanalysis. It is difficult to estimate to what extent the advisory from Varga was informed by his early engagement with psychoanalysis. For researchers to separate genuine engagement from obligatory, when it comes to materials produced at that time, is quite a complicated task, and to see the actual impact of psychoanalysis on political scene is even less possible.

As Gilgen argues, though, Marxism was not seen as a dogma, "but as a system of theoretical perspectives" (Gilgen, 1997, p. 5). Theoretical diversity of psychology was one of the features of the post-revolutionary period. "Empirical psychology, behavioural psychology (as manifested in reactology and reflexology), and psychoanalysis coexisted with various socially oriented fields of psychology" (Gilgen, 1997, p. 4). This mixture did not avoid psychoanalysis. A problem with the combination of psychoanalysis and Marxism was raised in 1922 in one of the meetings of the Kazan club. It was stated that "Marx and Freud: 1) both are analytical through and through; 2) both are concerned with the human unconscious; 3) the object of both methods is the personality in its social and historical context; 4) both study dynamics'" (Etkind, 1997, p. 228). This combination received the name 'Freudomarxism', however, as a project it failed to continue existing later than the 1930s, when to put it in one phrase: combining Marx with Freud became a crime.

In reality, it is difficult to evaluate the extent of the engagement of psychoanalysis and Marxism in Soviet Russia in the 1920s and 1930s due to the rapid changes in the political climate. After the Revolution, the early 20s were full of hope for a prosperous future, both in society and in the sciences. In his memoires, Luria shared that he was among many scientists who genuinely supported the Revolution and tried to engage with the writings of Marx and Lenin in their own work. During the era of Stalin, ideological demands became violent and worsened each year. Referencing Marx and Lenin became an obligatory element for any scholarly writing. Considering these circumstances, the combination of psychoanalysis and Marxism does not appear unusual.

What had more influence on psychoanalysis is the Sovetization of science in general, which led to the appearance of new theories. Soviet psychology divided into several branches: pedology,[3] socio-cultural psychology, pathopsychology, psychotechnics, psychohygiene, reactology, defectology etc. After the prohibition of psychology in the 1930s, and the proclamation of reflexology as an official approach to science, physiology now had to absorb and take over topics and research related to psychology. New terminology appeared: 'higher nervous activity' substituted for 'conscious', 'set' for 'unconscious', etc. That shift in the terminology confused later researchers, who attributed those changes to the shift of personal interests of scholars rather than to the demands of the times. The reality was that, to avoid persecution, scientists often altered their terminology or were forced to develop a coded language for their writing.

It is interesting, however, that the suitability of psychoanalysis for Vygotsky and Luria, as Chukhrov notices, was that "Freud managed to emphasize the impact of pure biology and evade the psyche" (2020, p. 156). Here she refers to their preface to the Russian edition of Freud's *Beyond the Pleasure Principle* (1925). She continues:

> For the Soviet Marxists, psyche was some kind of euphemism for spiritualism. What they approved of in this work of Freud's is how the psyche is exceeded by broader biological procedures and is thus considered to be part of a larger realm of biological phenomena. Vygotsky claims that Freud's *todestrieb* (death drive) overcomes the libidinal principle of drive, unravelling in it a materialistic, biological angle.
> 
> (Chukhrov, 2020, p. 156)

Speaking more about Vygotsky and Voloshinov, however, she does not spend any more time on Luria's work. This note about the materiality of the psychoanalytic approach to psyche, its embodiment (I refer here to Freud's quote, "The Ego is always primarily a bodily Ego" (Freud, 1923, p. 26)) indeed proved to be a bridge. However, it is less likely that it had anything to do with the Marxist emphasis on materiality, than simply conveniently suiting the direction of the main party line.

Detailed discussion about Luria's role in combining psychoanalysis with Marxism can be found in the work of Proctor (2016, 2020). Proctor's study, it is important to emphasize, does not seek to perform "a post-mortem psychological assessment of historical actors. Neither does it seek to lament what did not come to pass, nor to speculate upon what might have been" (p. 157). For her, Luria's interest was never primarily psychoanalytic and reading Freud for him was always combined with "other psychological approaches and read it through a Marxist lens" (p. 157). Proctor concludes that Luria failed both Freud and Marx, as his own research ignored social and historical circumstances of the participants of his studies (p. 177).

The eclectic nature of Luria and Vygotsky's studies is something that is usually used as an argument against their psychoanalytic affinity. The fact that someone reads and engages with philosophers or is in a dialogue with neurologists does not make him or her less psychoanalytically oriented. We would expect quite the opposite, looking at Freud, whose fascination with various views on the mind and human nature – from neurology to numerology – was constant throughout all his life.

Overall, it does not look like the engagement with Marxism was a specific feature of the Soviet followers of psychoanalysis or had much impact on the destiny of psychoanalysis in the USSR. It is not because of its engagement with Marxism that psychoanalysis failed to stay in the vanguard of psychology.

### The lack of clinical development

In his book on the history of psychoanalysis in Russia, Dmitry Rozhdestvenskii claims that in the early period, that is the 1920s, psychoanalysis lacked a clinical perspective (Rozhdestvenskii, 2009, p. 95). Most of the studies, he argues, were cultural and authors tried to imply that psychoanalysis was a form of worldview. As a result, he suggests, engagement with psychoanalysis in the early Soviet era remained superficial. So that is why it was so easy for Soviet scientists to recant psychoanalysis in the 1930s.

My first objection to this would be a reminder that psychoanalysis is not a purely clinical method. Therefore, it is precisely because Russian psychiatrists did not treat psychoanalysis as a strictly clinical method that I believe it demonstrates an ability for wider thinking, like contemporary psychosocial studies. Psychoanalytic theory, rather than the strictly clinical method of psychoanalysis, enhanced ideas developed in psychology and physiology and kept psychoanalysis 'live' beyond 1930. Continuing to develop the argument on the neglect of the clinical side of psychoanalysis, Rozhdestvenskii suggests that a contempt for neuroses as a bourgeois illness was a legitimate reason for the absence of clinical development in psychoanalysis after the 1920s (Rozhdestvenskii, 2009, p. 97) That is to say, there would not be a place for neuroses in socialist society, and therefore, no need for practices to treat them.[4]

When it comes to the actual lack of clinical perspective, it is still difficult to agree with Rozhdestvenskii. A pioneer of Russian psychoanalysis, Nikolay Osipov, brought psychoanalysis into the medical field. He was a psychiatrist and "celebrated the new therapeutic orientation which Freud was pursuing and felt that this method was important enough to be brought to the immediate attention of the psychiatric community in Russia". He visited Freud in Vienna and later sent to him two prints of his original writings, which Freud mentioned in a letter to Jung (Miller, 1998, p. 27).

Nikolay Vyrubov, professor of medicine, and Moshe Wulff, who studied and practiced in Berlin and later become an analysand of Karl Abraham (Miller, 1998, pp. 32–33) and returned to Russian Empire to work with patients, were both interested in the clinical application of psychoanalysis. Vyrubov and Osipov established a journal on Psychotherapy [*Psikhoterapiia*], the editorial board of which was later joined by psychiatrists Asatiani, A.N. Berstein and Iu.B. Kannabikh (Miller, 1998, p. 34). Another psychiatrist,

Tatiana Rosental, joined the psychoanalytic movement and brought it to Saint-Petersburg (Etkind, 1997, pp. 189–190). The years 1922–1928 were marked by another surge of activity in publishing. At that time, a new series, *The Psychological and Psychoanalytic Library*, [*Psikhologicheskaia and Psikhoanaliticheskaia Biblioteka*] in the State Publishing House [Gosizdatelstvo] under the editorship of Ivan Ermakov, published a series of translations of Freud, Jung, Abraham, Jones, Tausk, Ferenzi, Klein and other psychoanalysts. All that clinical activity echoed through later years and impacted the activity of the Bekhterev Psychoneurological Institute in Saint-Petersburg (where Rosental practiced). Founded in 1907, this Institute from the beginning was a research centre, a hospital, and a study centre where psychiatrists and neurologists could enhance their knowledge and skills in new approaches to mental health treatments. A founder of the Leningrad school of psychotherapy, Miasishchev,[5] studied psychoanalysis and supported Freud's claim regarding sexual trauma as a cause for neurosis. He developed his own concept of neuroses and approach to psychotherapy, which even today constitutes practice in the Bekhterev Psychoneurological Institute, where he was a director from 1939. Angelini (1988) suggests that Miasischev's practice was influenced by psychoanalysis.

Yes, there was plenty of interest in topics outside the clinic among clinicians. Osipov analysed Tolstoy's writings (Miller, 1998, p. 37) and Rosental analysed Dostoevsky's[6] and many more – according to information given by Ovacharenko in three first volumes of his *Summary of Psychoanalysis*. But this was not a Russian invention at all, not a specific Russian feature, neither it is presented as a clinical development. Freud's interest in the analysis of literature and art, his analysis of everyday life – jokes, slips of the tongue, and dreams – have always been an important part of psychoanalysis and deepened the clinical method.

Rozhdestvenskii noticed that members of the institute of the Russian Psychoanalytic Society organized by Ermakov in 1922 were not solely medical specialists. Its members included a professor of literature, a professor of mathematics, a professor of art and aesthetic studies, and a professor of physics (Rozhdestvenskii, 2009, p. 92). For Rozhdestvenskii, this indicated a superficial acceptance of psychoanalysis. Miller also mentions the same concern on behalf of the IPA organization towards Russia. In 1922 at the IPA Congress in Berlin, concerns were raised about the fact that a lot of members of the Moscow and Kazan groups were not doctors.

> The idea that a mathematician (Otto Shmidt) was the vice president of the Moscow Institute was inexplicable to medical people. The IPA also did not put much emphasis at this time on research in applied psychoanalysis by scholars in social psychology, philosophy, aesthetics, or history, fields in which the Russian were already making contributions.
> (Miller, 1998, p. 61)

However, Freud himself voted in 1924 for the acceptance of the Russian group. We know that Freud, in the text *The Question of Lay Analysis* (1926), formulated his view that a psychoanalyst need not be a medical doctor. He concluded that to be a psychoanalyst, one must be in analysis oneself and be familiar with psychoanalytic theory. He did not see a medical education as necessary for a psychoanalyst.

Continuing his arguments on the superficiality of the acceptance of psychoanalysis, it was important for Rozhdestvenskii that Luria came into psychoanalysis as a student of the faculty of law of Kazan University, and his initial interest was sociology (Rozhdestvenskii, 2009, p. 94). That amends a great period of Luria's interest in experimental studies of psychoanalysis and his further semi-forced turn to medicine. In 1937, Luria graduated from the 1$^{st}$ Moscow Medical University, and later became well known as a founder of Soviet neuropsychology – the hybrid of ideas derived from Luria's early interest in psychoanalysis and physiology, as further chapters of this book will argue. Although Luria was widely recognized for his studies of aphasia, memory, and brain functions, he also contributed to psychopathology – a branch of clinical psychology concerned with diagnosis and treatment of mental disturbances, established by Zeigarnik. Luria is an example of how psychoanalysis transformed and impacted the career and interests of one person, more than Rozhdestvenskii suggests.

Etkind's study supports the following line of the interpretation:

> At the State Psychoanalytic Institute, Spielrein gave a course on the psychology of unconscious thought and a seminar on child psychoanalysis. At a meeting of the Russian Psychoanalytic society in November 1923, she read a paper entitled 'Aphasic and Infantile Thought,' in which she asserted that the disruption of thought process in cases of aphasia was similar to children's thoughts, and both of these types of thought shed light on the process of speech formation.... Spielrein was working in the institute at just the time when Vygotsky was cutting a swath for himself in a field that was new for him.... The intellectual interests and development of talented people can be set for a long time to come by impressions gleaned at the very beginning of their careers from contact with a bright, famous, productive figure. Vygotsky's acquaintance with Spielrein could have played just such a role in the formation of his psychological interests.
>
> (Etkind, 1997, pp. 171, 173, 174)

One more contradiction I find difficult to accept in Rozhdestvenskii's argument on the superficiality of acceptance of psychoanalysis is his own reference to Dostoevsky. Rozhdestvenskii remarks that Dostoevsky anticipated the main psychoanalytic findings on human nature. For example, Ivan Karamazov exclaims before a court: "Who of us didn't want to kill his father?" Netochka Nezvanova says ("a half-century before the concept of child sexuality appeared" – emphasizes Rozhdestvenskii): "And since that minute some kind of limitless love to my father appeared in me, but wonderful love and not a child love at all" and later she shares her fantasies "When my mother will die, my father will leave this boring apartment and will go somewhere new with me" (Rozhdestvenskii, 2009, pp. 42–43). And that is only a little piece of a wide range of examples we can find in Dostoevsky, who prepared his readers for the acceptance of psychoanalytic ideas.

Paradoxically, after the chapter on the openness of the Russian scientific society towards psychoanalysis, and regarding the particular qualities of culture and literature that paved the way for Freud, Rozhdestvenskii concludes that the perception of psychoanalysis was superficial, not clinical, and that was the reason for its abandonment in the 1930s. For him, political reasons were not sufficient. He writes,

> Psychoanalysis never was officially prohibited, the ban on it existed behind the scenes. Ermakov, whose death is usually used as a piece of evidence to support the purges against psychoanalysis was arrested by NKVD not for being a psychoanalyst, but for anti-Soviet agitation activity. Most of the former psychoanalysts in the 1930s *simply trained for a new profession*, pedologists, physiologists, psychologists.
> (Rozhdestvenskii, 2009, p. 118, my emphasis)

Given that a lot of people died and disappeared in purges at the time, claiming that it was simply because psychoanalysts *decided* to change their professions is not convincing.

Another reason, which is never discussed as possibly facilitating evasive attitudes towards psychoanalysis, is the question of sexuality. As Rozhdestvenskii and Roudinesco noted, the role of libidinal forces tends to be ignored, and we can see the attempt to concentrate on sublimation instead.[7] In the early period of the 1920s, that focus on sublimation might happen because of the 'biological' critique of Freud. At first, he was criticized for emphasizing libidinal forces too much, and that contradicted the general line of the Party. After the shift in psychology in the 1930s and Pavlov's Session in 1950, all social reasoning gradually became prohibited and biological factors came to the front. The critique of Freud was no longer concerned with biology but was applied mostly to the idealistic nature of his ideas as opposed to materialism and its Western origin. The reason for sexuality vanishing from Soviet psychology was, nevertheless, more connected with the gradual shift in social policies towards sexuality that will be discussed further.

In fact, before the October Revolution of 1917 and the establishment of the Soviet Union, psychoanalysis was predominantly the interest of psychiatrists, who searched for new ways of treatment. In the 1920s, it expanded to the non-clinical field and led to the engagement of psychoanalysis with literature, cultural studies, and more importantly with Marxism.[8] However, "for the psychoanalytic community, these new conditions provided an enormous challenge. Survival was not possible without the approval and tolerance of the party" (Miller, 1998, p. 54). Under the pressure of the new State, everything in Russia had to be transformed according to the general plan of Union development that included not only economic rebuilding, but social and ideological transformation from the old tsarist regime to the socialist state.

Although roughness of the time for Russian psychoanalysis in the 1930s is acknowledged (Kozulin, 1984; Roudinesco, 1990; Etkind, 1997; Miller, 1998; Rozhdestvenskii, 2009), there is no further analysis to as why. The series of attacks on Freud in the mid-1920s, the suspension of psychoanalytic activities and the changes in the careers of prominent followers of psychoanalysis are not linked to the changes brought by the gradual rise of Stalinism to science in general (Krementsov, 1996; Pollock, 2006). Psychoanalysis did not escape the fate of the diverse 'psychologies' that got reduced to the new Soviet psychology, cleared from any foreign, bourgeois or reactionary ideas (Fraser and Yasnitsky, 2015). Although some unofficial activities around Freud's name were present between 1930 and 1980, in the current historical narrative they were seen mostly as critical of the place of psychoanalysis in Soviet psychology, regarding it as 'abandoned' theory (Pollock, 1982; Etkind, 1997; Miller, 1998; Rozhdestvenskii, 2009; Proctor, 2020). Some authors, however, see psychoanalysis as not having completely disappeared from the psychological scene, but rather remaining present under the cover of quasi-criticism (Kozulin, 1984; Angelini, 2008; Yasnitsky, 2009), as evidenced in memoirs of that time (Shoshin, 1992; Arnold, 1999; Kadyrov, 2005; Rotenberg, 2015; Mazin, 2018). Psychoanalytic methods were also occasionally adopted in clinical practice by psychiatrists (Rotenberg, 2015; Zajicek, 2009).[9]

## Negated psychoanalysis

Now with the socio-historical circumstances in mind, and knowing the general shifts in science under Stalin and in psychology in particular, we can try again to answer the question 'what had really happened with psychoanalysis in the Soviet Union?' Was it really the dissolution of psychoanalysis or rather a compulsory transformation? The short answer to this is – both.

In the article 'History of the Unconscious in Soviet Russia: From its origins to the fall of the Soviet Union' (2008) which explores how the concept of the unconscious and psychoanalysis was treated in Russia between 1900 and 1991 Angelini suggests that psychoanalysis was repressed rather than disappearing – an important emphasis of the forced nature of the turn 'away' from psychoanalysis. Starting with the early years of the 20th century, Angelini describes the atmosphere in Russia according to the tradition established by Etkind and Miller. The interpretations of the events that happened in psychoanalysis in Russia among these authors are more or less in accordance with each other and repeat the same chain of events. Etkind, Miller and

Angelini agree that psychoanalytic ideas flourished in Russia before the Revolution of 1917: it was supported by the political regime, it was mixed with Marxism or there were attempts to do so, it was "divorced from the clinical practice" but nevertheless widespread. Repetition of these ideas about psychoanalysis can only lead to the conclusion – which is repetition itself – that psychoanalysis was not compatible with Soviet state ideology and thus disappeared after the official ban. The main figures of the psychoanalytic movement either died, were killed, or emigrated. The political climate from the second half of the 1930s claimed to leave no one to support the psychoanalytic movement: "Soviet repression became so violent and all – encompassing that it struck not only the psychoanalytic movement, but even its adversaries. In other words, the concept of the unconscious could not be mentioned, not even in criticism" (Angelini, 2008, p. 376). According to Angelini, it was the Soviet government that repressed psychoanalysis between the years of 1930 and 1958. The fall of the Soviet Union, Angelini suggests, opened in the history of the unconscious in Russia a new chapter, "the return of the repressed".

The repression, in my view, was not as effective as Angelini suggests. Even in early days of the repression we find multiple examples of publications about Freud, psychoanalysis and 'Freudism'. Following the mention made by Miller of the article on psychoanalysis published in 1933 in *The Soviet Medical Encyclopaedia*, one of the authoritative scientific sources of that time, written by V. Vnukov and showing respect for some Freudian ideas, I've found out that several more articles dedicated to Freud, psychoanalysis and Freudism appeared in different volumes of Soviet Encyclopaedias throughout the period of 1930–1980.

The first edition of *The Small Soviet Encyclopaedia* in 1930 (vol. 7, p. 20) had an article about psychoanalysis, written by Yurii Kannabikh, who values the clinical efficacy of psychoanalysis, but stands against generalising its principle to phenomena outside the clinic. Articles on Freud and Freudism appeared in the next volume of *The Small Soviet Encyclopaedia* in 1931 (vol. 9, pp. 484–488) with, however, a radical change of tone. Their author, L. Shvartz, accuses Freud of being an idealistic thinker, and Freudism as being a profoundly reactionary theory. In 1939 the second edition of *The Small Soviet Encyclopaedia* did not have an article about psychoanalysis. However, in the first edition of *The Great Soviet Encyclopaedia*, 1940 (vol. 47), one of the most authoritative sources in the Soviet Union in general, we find an article on psychoanalysis, written by Alexander Luria. In 1947, in the second edition of *The Small Soviet Encyclopaedia* (vol. 11, pp. 362–363) there is no article about Freud, but an article about Freudism as pseudo-scientific theory remains. In the second edition of *The Great Soviet Encyclopaedia* in 1956 (vol. 35, p. 237 and vol. 45, pp. 583–584) there are articles on psychoanalysis, Freud and Freudism. They are much shorter, and with no author's signature. In 1967, *The Encyclopaedia of Philosophy* (vol. 4, pp. 417–419) contained an article on psychoanalysis and in 1970 (vol. 5, pp. 410–412, 412–414) articles on Freud and Freudism. The third edition of the *The Great Soviet Encyclopaedia* in 1975 (vol. 21, pp. 187–188) appeared with the article about psychoanalysis, and in 1978 (vol. 28, p. 85) with the article about Freudism.

Basically, there was only one volume, in 1939, which excluded psychoanalysis from the encyclopaedia. Otherwise, volumes and editions kept articles on Freud and Freudism through all the years. Growing up in the Soviet Union, anyone will recognize the covers of *Soviet Encyclopaedias*, which were a must in the home library of the general citizen. Knowledge of the existence of Freud and psychoanalysis was surely available to anyone.[10]

However, the fact that it was included there, and the words unconscious and psychoanalysis were still mentioned twice after its ban in 1930, opens the door for investigation. A brief search of titles and content in the Russian State Library during that period resulted in 286 articles and books containing references to psychoanalysis between 1930 and 1950. The list is not complete, but it shows the presence of an interest in psychoanalysis even in times of the ban. Further chapters of this book will elaborate on the presence of psychoanalysis in both public and academic discussions.

To use a term, 'negation', I argue, would better describe the situation. While negation is a form of repression, it is a failed repression. As Freud (1925a) writes, it consists of the affirmation and the negative particle 'no'. Its function is to keep the unpleasant thought out of consciousness by rejecting it in language. The phrase "we do not have psychoanalysis in the USSR" should be read as "we do have psychoanalysis in the USSR, but we are having trouble with it". For Freud, negation is not bad for our psychic functioning. Unlike repression, it does not exclude presentations from consciousness and therefore we can still be aware of objects, but in a negated form. Moreover, these negated presentations can be used for our thinking and that's how the subject could develop knowledge about unpleasant events and objects. Conversely, repressed presentations are excluded from the thinking process, and they also exclude presentations connected with unpleasant experiences by associative links (Freud, 1925a).

Repressed psychoanalysis would not affect the thinking of Soviet scientists and could only re-emerge at some point, while negated psychoanalysis would be constantly present and could circulate in thinking. In my view, this is what possibly happened. Of course, if Angelini uses the notion of repression not in a psychoanalytic sense, but with reference to Stalin's repressions, in which anything not in accordance with the view of the Party should have been demolished – it totally makes sense. Psychoanalysis was under repression, went underground, and then was rehabilitated after Stalin's death. However, while real political rehabilitation happened only in 1996, when President Boris Yeltsin signed the official decree 'On the Revival and Development of Philosophical, Clinical and Applied Psychoanalysis', the discussion around Freud was rehabilitated much earlier, in 1958 during the Freud Session.

In the socio-historical context, as we have seen, negation also played an important role in constructing the responses to the pressure of ideology.

Moreover, negation opens the room for a more nuanced understanding of the vicissitudes of psychoanalysis in the field of Soviet science under the pressure of Stalinism and after. To understand where the negation is coming from, we need to investigate the changes in the language milieu as it constituted conditions and opportunities for survival, both scientifically and in everyday life, and return to the notion of splitting.

## A language "affair": The new scientific language in the Soviet Union 1930–1980

The language of the Party leaders – Stalin, Khrushchev and Brezhnev – whose speeches dictated the direction of the country's development, constituted an important determinant of for the direction of everyday life and science between the late 1920s and 1980. Being a component of the authoritative discourse in science, the new academic language mirrored the language set by the party members. The shift in the scientific language of Soviet psychology and physiology, which began in the late 1920s, peaked in the 1950s at the infamous Pavlov Session.

Krementsov points out that this language was one of the three major components of the social practice of Soviet scientists distinctive to Stalinist science. The other two were public behaviour and styles of criticism (Krementsov, 1996, p. 6). The importance of the scientific style in writings and speech is not something unusual; of course, it was significant in determining how scientists expressed their ideas long before the Soviet regime. However, during Soviet times the style of language adopted by scientists held extra meaning and importance because it was a major component of social practice. I suggest seeing Soviet language as a part of the living conditions that structured the way in which things were done and lives were lived. In other words, language created the effective milieu for all Soviet citizens, including academics. So, a scientific language emerged as a response to the general shift in language milieu and it was constantly transforming throughout 1930–1980.

As a recently-emerged state, the USSR had to be built economically, ideologically, scientifically, and socially. By the time Stalin became General Secretary (1922) it was almost certain that international revolution would not happen and, therefore, resources for the building of a new state should be taken from inside. Soviet language played an important role very early on and was changed specifically due to the need for the consolidation of all the population. Agit-prop posters, newspapers and speeches of the party leaders covered by slogans were widely distributed and became a part of the environment. Something we now address as the aesthetics of the Soviet Union was a condition of life for millions of people. Further, alongside industrialization of the country and the First Five-Year Plan implementation (1928), a plan to transform the being of Soviet citizens, including the mind, was executed on many layers of life. Introduction of *novyi byt* and *kulturnost* introduced trends in how an individual should live in the socialist regime, leisure, health habits, and fashion and consumption. New language entered the cinema, literature, and art. The State was addressing its individuals basically everywhere. This very specific milieu for citizens was supposed to bring a feeling of identity with the new values of socialism. The expectation of prosperity became an important part of the narrative, which also emphasized the value of individual contributions to the collective. To be proud of citizenship and to be ready to sacrifice for citizenship made the experience of being Soviet. Prosperity, however, was placed in the future. In psychoanalytic terms, the future had to be *idealized* to sustain being in the present.

On the other hand, civil war, famine, the rise of crime, purges, the violence of the 1920s brought destruction, disruption and left many lives in ruin. Daily life was far from satisfying. As Fitzpatrick notes (1999, p. 165) 'normal' life at that time was an 'ideal', and 'living normally' meant living a privileged life that most people did not have. By the time of the end of the First Five-Year Plan (1932), living conditions did not improve and the country was still in devastation. Living conditions for many were below the poverty line. Urbanization went not as fast as required, and while many people left the countryside to work in cities, it created housing shortages. Quite a common form of housing was so-called *kommunalka* 'communal flats'. Normally it was an apartment with no less than five rooms, (sometimes up to ten), with one bathroom and one kitchen shared between all residents. So, several families with children co- habited with other families and individuals. Privacy was impossible, and a queue to the bathroom or the toilet was normal.[11] People lived with shortages of clothes, household essentials, food, and much else. The life of academics was not an exception, although it is rarely mentioned that they also had to live through famine, shortages, deprivation of essential goods etc. The purges that continued in the 1930s, and then again in the 1950s added to this hardship; fear and uncertainty flourished. The life of academics, again, was not an exception. The threat of arrest, for example, was present for Luria and Zeigarnik throughout the late 1930s, 1940s and even 1950s (Cole, Levitin, and Luria, 2014; Zeigarnik, 2001).

Party leaders contributed to this splitting not only through the political agenda. The split was supported on several levels. Their *public behaviour* sustained a special image for each of them. Being presented as Great Fathers of the USSR, they combined sublime and very human qualities. Even though Stalin's time is described as a cult of personality, not many of his personal features were known to the public. Instead, his personality was substituted by the image, which eventually became a symbol. Mass production of Stalin's portraits and statues made him omnipresent. The discourse of family relationships substituted for comradeship and made Stalin as close as a family member, changing the common way of addressing relationships between citizens. Everyone became brothers and sisters, under Father Stalin and Mother Land. Every man became an 'uncle', every woman became an 'aunt' to a stranger (Brandenberger, 2005; Perrie, 2001; Plamper, 2012).

There were other changes as well, that constituted the 'environment' of the state even more. For example, Stalin's vocabulary was filled with words and expressions he invented himself. A study by Mikhail Weiskopf dedicated to the language of Stalin and his literary talent begins with "Stalin edited the USSR. At the same time, he created the main text for his state" (Weiskopf, 2001, p. 7). Of course, one can say that the Russian language was not native to Stalin, and his use of language was often beyond the grammatical rules because of that. Exotic use of words outside their usual meanings, sexual connotations, the motive of struggle, absurdity combined with clarity and accessibility of his speeches to the mass, this is just a short list of qualities Weiskopf attributes to Stalin's language. A good example of ambivalence might be his phrase, used regularly in speeches, "Friendly fight with enemies" (Weiskopf, 2001, p. 24). However, it was not only about the language he used, but the reality that was created by this language. Or, rather, the great transformation of reality that started there and the creation of the new environment that continued through many years of Soviet leadership.

Inhabiting the borderline between comedy and tragedy, eccentric elements were common features of the speeches of the Soviet leaders after Stalin also. Their language and expressions became the source for anecdotes, jokes and stable expressions. Let's look at Khrushchev's phrase "we shall show you Kuzka's mother" addressed to President Nixon, that is deeply grounded in the language, even nowadays. On the level of meaning, this is an expression of a threat to someone and a promise of punishment, while its linguistic form is ironic and has the tone of a joke. Unusual gestures, loose language, curious and embarrassing situations were part of Khrushchev's image. It is not surprising that the rumour that in the United Nations General Assembly meeting in New York in October 1960 he took off his shoe and banged the desk with it stays in the narrative around him, although it was never documented as a historical fact. It captures something important about Khrushchev's behaviour and presentation, as well as his policies. His campaign of de-Stalinization that aimed to bring clarity and truth about Stalin's era, additionally split society. As Jones (2006) indicates, freedom of expression of criticism towards Stalin was both encouraged and controlled, and eventually "dissenting voices were silenced more forcefully" (p. 59). Moreover, Reich (2018) shows how Khrushchev sanctioned the use of psychiatric diagnosis in the persecution of dissenters, which opened the era of psychiatric abuse and collaborations with the state. Freedom of thought was only allowed when thoughts were in line with the general party line.

Khrushchev's successor, Brezhnev, who ruled the country from 1964 to his death in 1982, continued to support the established tradition of ambiguity. Despite Brezhnev calling this time 'developed socialism', the economy, social life and politics were in continuous crisis, leading to the period up to 1987 being known as the Era of Stagnation. While both views are supported historically (Suny, 2011) and represent the complexity of that period, they also show the discord between the 'official' and 'real' situations. No wonder that many Soviet citizens started to experience even more difficulties with accepting the idea of the superiority of the USSR. Brezhnev's public behaviour, although being more 'adequate' in comparison with Stalin or Khrushchev, was also not without eccentric gestures. His famous habit of giving kisses on lips during political meetings immortalized him on the famous graffiti on the east side of the Berlin wall (*My God Help Me to Survive This Fatal Attraction*, or The Kiss, author Dmitri Vrubel, 1990). The way young Brezhnev presented his ideas and his language was stuffed with jokes; he is known for eccentric acts while meeting with Western leaders. His publicly known passion was to drive cars given to him by representatives of world countries and to exceed the speed limit. In his later years, his speeches were known to be very slow and hypnotic, due to his progressive illness and addiction, but not without with the humorous aspect to it. Perhaps he is best known for making great jokes and using humour as a constant component of his political interactions, but also, he is the most famous figure of jokes himself. At the same time, during the Brezhnev period, Soviet psychiatry entered the peak of the era of abuse and persecution of dissents. It was the time of the spread of the phenomenon of 'internal emigration', a very specific defence Soviet citizens developed, which "captures precisely the state of being inside and outside at the same time, the inherent ambivalence of this oscillating position" (Yurchak, 2005, p. 142).

With their ambivalent policies, public appearance and gestures, by presenting themselves as close to ordinary humans, at the same time holding onto the façade of Soviet pride and greatness and denying state crimes and their personal contribution to the purges, abuse, etc., the great party leaders contributed to the establishment of the split society. Denial of the 'bad' parts of the country's life they created served their own interests. By proclaiming Stalin's mistakes, Khrushchev covered up his own restrictive policies, while Brezhnev totally denied the presence of problems. Their *language* and the rhetoric they used set up the environment of the denial for the entire country.

The country ended living in several dimensions at once, which is very well captured in a joke about the confusion of a man who watched TV and saw the great country USSR there, and then looked out of the window and couldn't find it. From the psychoanalytic point of view, the effect this split had not only on living conditions, but also on the sense of being and identity, must have been tremendous.

The idealization of the state thickened under the need for sacrifice during the Great Patriotic War, coinciding with the Third Five-Year Plan (1938–1942). The polarity was intensified through the figure of the enemy, the German invader, attacking Mother Russia. The negation of war losses, violence within the army, the negative impact of war on the economy etc. came alongside the idealization of the victory and the great defence of the motherland. The historical continuity that was created by propaganda just before the war brought into public discourse the figures of Alexander Nevsky and Ivan Grozny – great defenders of the Medieval Rus. That also thickened national ideas of Russian greatness (Perrie, 2001; Pollock, 2006). The idea of the multicultural state USSR and friendship of all nations under the umbrella of socialism was lost and, instead, society got homogenized under the Russian banner.

The same processes were mirrored in academia. The new language and the work of splitting gradually also affected it. The movement towards a new science went along with Collectivization (started in 1928). As Graham points out, these were years when the Academy of Sciences and the universities were purged and reorganized. Most of the damage fell on the social sciences, although the natural sciences did not stay untouched. The shift especially happened in the year of 'the Great Break' (1928–1929), "before that date the contents of the journals are heterogeneous in outlook, and genuine intellectual controversies occur. After 1929 the journals become thinner and a veil of orthodoxy is pulled over all discussions" (Graham, 1993, p. 120). Discussions were not any more concerned about the content of academic papers, but with their ideological appearance. So, it was logical to see how policies began to dominate ideas, and how changes were determined by administrators, rather than scientists themselves. "The granting of higher degrees, personnel assignment and promotion, scientific publishing, academic research and instruction – all were subject to the control of Party officials" (p. 121). The system of censorship operated on multiple layers, from academic publications to secondary school textbooks. Top positions in academia, publishing and research were appointed by the central Party organs. This, argues Graham, is why it was possible by 1948 to give such ideas as Lysenko's monopolistic status, "despite the opposition of established geneticists" (p. 121) – and, I would add, despite common sense.

In the period of the immediate post-war years and the Fifth Five-Year Plan (1946–1950), we find examples not only of the work of negation and splitting, but also the emergence of many unrealistic ideas. This is in accordance with the psychoanalytic view on the consequences of the splitting. For Melanie Klein, the mental mechanism of splitting led to the division into the bad object, which is demonized, and the good object, which is idealized. The process of idealization, according to Klein, has dangerous results for the mind, because the idealized object is separated from the rule of reality and operates according to the logic of fantasy. In other words, idealization creates unrealistic objects and unrealistic ideas. They can follow wishful thinking, or they can just depart from reality into made-up worlds. While of course we are thinking about not a mind, but a society, the operational logic of paranoid-schizoid position cannot be entirely applied here.

This is the one way, however, to understand how it was possible to be serious about the findings of some Soviet scientists in this decade. Examples of such idealistic ideas can be found in the work of biologist Lepeshinskaya (1945) who experimentally recreated the moment of transformation of inanimate matter into living matter, discussed at length in a book, *The Origin of*

*Cells From Living Matter and the Part Played by Living Matter in the Organism*. Of course, real science continued to be developed; however, the emergence of the unrealistic discoveries illustrates how the split between reality and fantasy, created by Stalin's megalomanic effort to transform society, was reproduced at many levels.

A better-known and more serious in its consequences example of idealization in science can be the movement of Lysenkoism or the so-called 'Lysenko affair', an attack on genetics in the Soviet Union in the period mid-1930s to mid-1960s with the domination of the unrealistic ideas of Lysenko and as a consequence devastation of agriculture in the USSR. As Pollock explains in the *Stalin and the Soviet Science Wars*, in the late 1940s "the 'West' supplanted the 'bourgeoisie' as the enemy; creating Soviet science, not proletarian science, became the goal" (Pollock, 2006, p. 104). To do so, Party leaders had to find and use 'homegrown trailblazers' for each scientific field, who would be in tune with the ideology. For example, in genetics, this scheme worked as such: Lysenko took the ideas of biologist Michurin and applied it in a pseudo-scientific way, creating a Michurin's biology, which was far away from the original work of Michurin. However, Michurin died in 1935, so he could not intervene.

The field of psychology did not avoid the transformations described above. Since the socialist society built by Stalin was seen as the ideal state with amazing conditions for its citizens, any impact on society apart from happy impacts had to be eradicated. This was one of the points of the decree of VKP(b) Central Committee "On Pedological Perversions in the System of Narkomproses" in 1936. It accused 'pedologists' of using "pseudoscientific experiments and harmful questionnaires to instil a belief in biosocial determinism" (Byford, 2020, p. 249). Through this decree, authorities prevented scientists developing social theories regarding children's development. After that, psychology underwent a huge transformation as a discipline and formed what was called Soviet psychology.[12] Terminologically, physiology 'hosted' psychologists, who now had to undertake research on 'consciousness' and 'higher nervous activity' and later 'higher nervous functions' which were the biologically terminological equivalent of the psyche. For many years, core research questions for psychologists were about temperament, types of nervous system, and the psychology of emotions and activity. The study of cognitive processes dominated the study of the individual as a whole.[13]

Even though psychology was not in the list of six major sciences participating in Stalin's 'science wars' – linguistics, genetics, physiology, political economy, philosophy and physics (Pollock, 2006) – changes around them affected psychology indirectly. The Joint Scientific Session of the USSR Academy of Sciences and the USSR Medical Sciences Academy, or the Pavlov Session, in 1951, made physiologist Ivan Pavlov into that 'homegrown trailblazer', and because he died in 1936 his work could be used in any useful way for the Party leaders. Pollock also emphasizes the emergence of what he calls 'Russocentrism' (Pollock, 2006, p. 7): non-Russians could not serve as the basis for the new Soviet science. References to Freud or any Western author in Soviet psychology or physiology once again became outlawed.

Elizabeth Roudinesco catches this split in science when exploring the Stalinist era and a shift from social reasoning to the search for a biological source for psychological disturbances and hence the growing worship of Pavlov. She references the thought of Emile Baulieu, who "proclaimed his love of Marxism by explaining that psychoses had disappeared in the Soviet Union" (Roudinesco, 1990, p. 187). Of course, while ideologically it was important to support the idea of a utopian prosperous society, in reality, Soviet citizens suffered from acute stress and dissatisfaction with a failure to realize that utopia. A Soviet turn to physiology (and away from psychoanalysis) aimed to mask the insufficiency of the new regime:

> In the land of Stalin, it was indeed proclaimed that madness did not exist; but since the deranged, the crazed, the demented, the maladapted and the neurotic were as frequently visible as in the capitalist world, Pavlovianism was reactivated in order to prove that madness did not derive from social causes, but from an organic or physiological substrate; that dimension would have to be treated in 'Michurinian' fashion in order to transform the insane into worshippers of the Soviet paradise.
>
> (p. 187)

Within a few years, it became difficult for a Soviet psychologist to develop a psychosocial approach to research due to the country's ideological-political constraints. No wonder that this shift resulted in changes of titles too. For example, Luria became a neuropsychologist and shifted his research to brain studies. This addition of 'neuro-' illustrates the necessity to follow an official ideological direction. Masquerade was not a new technique, however. Sirotkina writes about the split between the name and the action being in use already in 1924: "Under the cover of new terminology, Kornilov employees continued to research previously chosen topics. Luria's reference to 'affective reactions' covered his interest in psychoanalysis with its 'affective complexes'" (Sirotkina and Smith, 2016, p. 24). That observation captures changes specific to psychoanalysis, as the attack on psychoanalytic vocabulary started much earlier, to which I will turn in the next chapter. Anything related to mention of the 'unconscious' immediately would call for suspicion and the label of 'idealist theory'. Until the Freud Session in 1958, discussion about 'the unconscious' was impossible; instead, it was the 'non-conscious' or physiological processes behind consciousness that were studied.

## Negation

Writing on the unconscious in what he calls totalitarian society, Michael Rustin emphasizes the concrete nature of thinking and inability to produce thought due to the absence of alternative versions of reality from consideration:

> The free expression and exchange of ideas in society is of psychological as well as political importance, since, through allowing the emergence of many 'third positions', it is the precondition of thinking and engagement with reality. Without differences and contradictions, there can be no generative thought.
>
> (Rustin, 2016, p. 229)

In addition to Rustin, I suggest that we can find one more way of thinking which operated in Soviet society, related to Freud's notion of negation. According to Freud, negation creates a symbol and frees the intellectual space from the effects of repression. "With the help of the symbol of negation, thinking frees itself from the restrictions of repression and enriches itself with material that is indispensable for its proper functioning" (Freud, 1925a, p. 236). One can think of something, without being touched by the thought and without associating this thought with oneself, in an abstract way. A good literary example of this is Ivan Ilych, a character in the story written by Tolstoy, who is coming to terms with his own death. His thinking there concerned the archetypal man, Caius, who was mortal, and whose death is explored at length in the mind of Ivan Ilyich without posing a danger to Ivan Ilyich, who in his mind remained immortal.[14]

This idea will explain the emergence of the phenomena captured by Waterlow, Yurchak, Ledeneva, Kozulin, and Krementsov as discordance between words and practice, official identities, and underground ones, as well as emergence of the 'third' space beyond the dichotomy of the official and underground. "Concealment was a normal condition of Soviet life", states Fitzpatrick (1999, p. 132). As many people could not identify either with agreement or opposition to the 'totalitarian' reality, they had to live what she calls a 'double life', split into an 'invented' public self and a 'real' private self (Fitzpatrick, 1999).[15]

I am interested in this development of the third position in the 'alternative reality' space in academia and I think of it as constituted through the negation of the 'totalitarian' reality, although different from its denial. Negation can operate alongside splitting by helping to support unpleasant parts of the experience in consciousness without frustration. Negation operates within language, and is made possible through negating particles, such as 'no'. For example, according to newspapers in the Soviet Union, there was no sex in the USSR, there was no unhappiness in the USSR, there was no bureaucracy in the USSR, there was no inequality in the USSR, and there was no anti-Semitism in the USSR etc.

The success of the Pavlov Session in the eradication of non-Russian, idealistic and bourgeois theories from the Soviet scientific field, however, was not permanent. In 1958, physiologists, psychiatrists and former psychologists came together to discuss how to fight Freudism. This event, already discussed above, was the Freud Session held at the initiative of the Presidium of the Academy of Medical Sciences of the USSR. Apparently, there was a need to do so, even after eight years of Pavlov's rule. As we have seen, through the lens of the notion of negation the content of the speech of every presenter in the whole session will start looking like an exchange of the latest news in the field of Western psychoanalysis.

Situated in the broader historical context, this session happened two years after the Khrushchev Secret Speech in February 1956, which at that time was not available to the public, nevertheless was sent out to the local authorities for discussion. A short version was released as Central Committee resolution 'On the Cult of Personality and Its Consequences' on 30 June 1956. After that, the process called de-Stalinization brought quite a lot of changes into society in the attempt to "emancipate the popular consciousness from the Stalin cult" (Jones, 2006, p. 41).

In science this turn to relative freedom resonated in gradual denunciation of previously appointed leaders. Pavlov was one of them. In 1962, there took place another important scientific session, dedicated to the philosophical aspects of the higher nervous activity. Bluma Zeigarnik summarizes this turn in her book on pathopsychology (translated into English as 'Abnormal psychology'):

> Owing to the erroneous interpretation of certain statements of Ivan Petrovich Pavlov, the view was disseminated that psychology was supposedly concerned with the description of subjective phenomena and that for causal explanation, it was necessary to look only to the physiology of higher nervous activity. As a result of these false views, psychological research in psychiatry began to be replaced by physiological research. As we know, these views were criticized at the 1962 All-Union Conference on Philosophical Issues in the Physiology of Higher Nervous Activity and Psychology. This conference, which was convened by the Academy of Sciences of the USSR, the Academy of Medicine of the USSR, and the Academy of Pedagogical Sciences of the RSFSR, resolved to condemn biologizing tendencies in the science of man. The resolution noted that, after the 1950 session, 'the wide dissemination of a negative attitude toward psychology entailed practical harm and methodological error as some scholars tried to reduce the subject matter of psychology to the physiology of higher nervous activity.' Measures for the development of medical psychology were discussed at this conference together with other problems.
>
> (Zeigarnik, 1972, pp. 14–15)

After that conference, it was possible again to talk about psychology without using physiological terms only and to study Western authors more openly. However, another split happened, and the 1960s are known for the tightening of the collaboration between some psychiatrists and party leaders, resulting in the widespread practice of the forced hospitalization of political dissidents and those who expressed views different to the main ideology. Abuse in psychiatry continued to exist throughout the years of the USSR and put a huge shadow over Soviet psychiatry in the West, not to mention the reputation of mental health practitioners for the public. That harmed the workers in psychiatry and psychology who stayed away from the abuse and from collaboration with the Party. For many years after, to search for the help of a psychiatrist or psychologist was, in the public perception, considered dangerous.

We will see how this impacted on Luria, Zeigarnik, Uznadze, and Bassin in further chapters and how each of them addressed these challenges in their career. Before that I would like to return to the language milieu and discuss how these changes resulted in lives of ordinary citizens in more detail.

## Practices of being Soviet: Paradoxes of dimensions of meanings

When writing about the phenomenon of *blat* (or an informal practice of favour), Ledeneva (1998) draws attention to specific features of Soviet society, emphasizing its subversive character. Even though informal practices are not the focus of my study, Ledeneva's summary of the subversive structure of Soviet society is useful for my research for many reasons.

It begins with a Russian phrase '*nel'zya, no mozhno*' (prohibited but possible), that "offers a summary understanding of Soviet society with its all-embracing restrictions and the labyrinth of possibilities around them" (Ledeneva, 1998, p. 1). This is the reality captured in language and at the same time an example of language constituting the reality and providing an unwritten rule, or even a system of navigation within the split society. The informal practices "enabled the Soviet system to function and made it tolerable, but also subverted it" (p. 3). This subversion, however, did not always represent the active position of the resistance. Many of the participants of Ledeneva's study referred to it as routine practice (p. 5). Others denied their part in *blat* and described it "in terms of friendship or mutual help in the case of personal involvement" (Ibid., p. 6), although calling it *blat* when practiced by others. Overall, many of respondents "claimed that they had nothing to do with *blat*" (p. 6) while describing clear examples of it in their life during the interviews. A practice of *blat*, therefore, was interwoven into the being of almost everyone, and became so usual, it was impossible to notice it without making a special effort to recognize it.

Ledeneva continues (p. 77) that due to its elaborated bureaucratic system, Soviet society operated in an atmosphere of uncertainty, and unwritten codes regulated reality. Rules were both accepted and avoided, each rule had its exception. To apply written rules 'where necessary' blurred boundaries of official laws and created freedom, at the same time this freedom could be any time restricted. So everyone lived under the pressure of 'suspended punishment', which intended to keep everyone under self-control.

> The popular version of the idea of suspended punishment was expressed in an anecdote about a person who happened to be sentenced to five-year imprisonment. He was not guilty and did not understand what he was accused of and it was explained to him that if he were guilty indeed he would be sentenced to 10 years.
>
> (p. 78)

The informal practices described by Ledeneva in that context can be seen as defence mechanisms emerging in the society under the pressure of ambiguity and aiming to provide solutions for living. That gives us more details of a picture of the double dimension that existed in Soviet society. In that dimension one could agree and disagree with the rules at the same time. That combination in psychoanalytic theory constitutes perfect conditions for anxiety and subsequent splitting.

A similar structure is described by Jonathan Waterlow (2018) in relation to the role of humour in Stalinist times. Surprisingly, in a period when a joke could land a citizen with a custodial sentence, anecdotes and jokes circulated widely. For Waterlow, such subversive behaviour by ordinary citizens provided a semblance of freedom and identification, even a form of support in times of hardship.

> Activities like telling political jokes, trading on the black market, and exchanging favours certainly meant breaking the rules in the Soviet 1930s, but in practice transgressions like these were more often workarounds – ways to solve problems and get by *within* the system, rather than attempts to destabilise or to confront it
>
> (Waterlow, 2018, p. 188)

Waterlow's work describes the social reality outside the binary division in the 1930s, where his study is situated. "We shouldn't interpret people's use of Bolshevik or Soviet terms to discredit officials or regime favourites as a sign that they were becoming trapped in it (and therefore somewhat subjugated by) official discourse or values, however" (Waterlow, 2018, p. 247). This is in agreement with Yurchak, who formulates how the mindset of

> late socialism [1960s-1980s] became marked by an explosion of various styles of living that were simultaneously inside and outside the system and can be characterized as *being vnye*. These styles of living generated multiple new temporalities, spatialities, social relations, and meanings that were not necessarily anticipated or controlled by the state, although they were fully made possible by it.
>
> (Yurchak, 2005, p. 128)

For example, the phrase *vne polia zreniia* (out of sight) is used when something is known to be here, but is invisible or obstructed from view by another object.

The operation Yurchack suggests here in my view is very close to the mechanism of disavowal, as it described by Freud, a specific form of negation where the negated object is not evacuated from the mind but declined. *Disavowal (Ger. Verleugnung)* ("I see that my mother has no penis, but I believe it is still there") is different from other forms of negation, such as *foreclosure* and *denial*. Freud uses this term to talk about castration in his work *Fetishism* (1927e), saying the subject accepts reality and disavows it at the same time. Moreover, affectively the subject continues to believe in the disavowed presentation (Freud, 1927e). According to Laplanche, Freud opposes this mechanism to repression, and later connect disavowal to fetishism. Freud also defines disavowal as the mechanism of denying an external reality (Laplanche and Pontalis, 1978).

At the same time, to disavow reality is not the same as to foreclose it. Freud adds another term – splitting (of ego) – to explain how disavowal could possibly operate. In foreclosure we find no symbolic sign about an object in the mental space, it is not affirmed, while in disavowal there is an affirmation and there is a sign about the object in the mental space, but on the level of action, the subject behaves as if there is no knowledge about it. This is possible through splitting on the level of ego as if one part of the ego recognizes reality, and the other does not. So, to put it briefly:

- in foreclosure representation is not created, the reality is ejected
- in denial representation is created, reality accepted with a symbolic 'no'
- in disavowal representation is created, the reality is ejected.

Disavowal works together with splitting. It is not the classic neurotic conflict between ego and id; this conflict is located between ego and reality.

Growing up in the Soviet Union, one should have developed the ability to hold the split between these dimensions. "But this didn't produce Orwell's infamous 'doublethink', in which two contradictory ideas are held hermetically sealed from each other in people's minds, never to interact. Nor did citizens develop a 'permanently schizophrenic vision' of the world and their lives" (Waterlow, 2018, p. 264). Psychoanalytically speaking, disavowal should have been the main mechanism operating to support this subversive order. This is not to claim that Soviet society was totally perverted in a clinical sense, but to see that the escape from a reality where everything was prohibited could actually exist through informal practices or humour, serving as well as mechanisms of defence against uncertainty, danger, shortages, censorship and many other sources of anxiety and frustration. That is formulated in a saying I frequently heard from my grandmother, which I put as an epigraph to this book: "If you really really want something, but it is prohibited, then it's allowed" (*Esli chego-to nelzia, no ochen hochetsia – to mozhno*).

## New ways of reading Soviet

It is only recently that re-examinations of Soviet psychology have shown that there existed informal connections between Soviet psychologists and their Western colleagues, and that international literature was available during the Soviet period, reinforcing the suggestion that Soviet-era psychologists were, in fact, highly erudite but operating at a time when subterfuge was necessary (Yasnitsky, 2012a). Thus, on one level the reality and ideology of the Stalinist era made it impossible to write freely. At the informal level a lot was possible, if it was conducted properly – that is, in secret or semi-secret (Kozulin, 1984, p. 89; Rotenberg, 2015, pp. 3–7). As a result, the fact that references to Western authors were either absent from or criticized in the printed works of Soviet psychologists did not mean that Western authors were not read, assimilated, and appreciated. If we look at the political campaign against psychoanalysis in particular, it can be maintained that Luria and Vygotsky were no different to their contemporaries, and we should question the nature of their criticism of psychoanalysis, especially when it appears in the 1930s.

After Khrushchev's secret speech in 1956, in medical science in general, and in psychology in particular, it became possible to address some Western authors. Consequently, having been previously outlawed, psychoanalysis and debates surrounding the existence and operation of the unconscious reappeared once more in official Soviet science. The discussion, however, was not an open one. A specific feature developed in the Soviet scientific field through the years of repression: a pseudo-critical style of writing. This feature affects our perspective on a whole heritage of thought.

> One and the same act – for example, a criticism of psychoanalysis – can be interpreted as a coincidence of the theoretical position of the author with accepted ideological clichés, as the fulfilment of an ideologically prescribed obligation, or even as a concealed method of propagation of psychoanalytical ideas that might otherwise have no chance of exposure.
> (Kozulin, 1984, p. 89)

An example of the discreet techniques Soviet academics used to deal with the Soviet prohibition on Western thought is the ground-breaking book on the unconscious written by Filipp Bassin (1968) who superficially presented a seemingly harsh critique of the notion of the unconscious 'from the Marxist standpoint', but by mere fact of this publication and its very detailed discussion of the literature on the unconscious, including the writings of Freud, reintroduced the problems of the unconscious to Soviet scientific discourse and initiated a discussion of psychoanalysis that had remained outlawed for several decades (Rotenberg, 2015; Savenko, 2005, 2006) (quoted by Yasnitsky, 2009, p. 109; and for the same conclusion see Mazin, 2018, pp. 43–44).

Yasnitsky proposes that the reader of Soviet writings must have a specific "set" towards it in order to understand it. Set as "the reader's or listener's orientation towards a specific semiotic system, and the implied rules of encoding it entails, is instrumental in adequately understanding Soviet scientific doublespeak" (Yasnitsky, 2009, p. 117). In this notion of set, Yasnitsky shares the same meaning as Jacobson's *Einstellung*. "Clearly, doublespeak poses considerable problems of 'retranslation', and much research needs to be done in conjunction by linguists, psychologists, and historians of culture and science, in order to decode The Code" (p. 117). In his dissertation he does semiotic and discursive research, defining such techniques of survival as *quasi-critique, shadowboxing, roles of laymen and spokesmen, specific referencing strategies, doublespeak*. For example, "Non-referencing became an instrument of survival and of continuing scientific research" (p. 106).

There is more to consider, beyond these distortions. Yasnitsky argues, "In contrast, the wide range of texts produced by Soviet scholars for publication or public presentation are relatively less reliable due to censorship and – even more importantly, self-censorship – in the Soviet Union from the early 1930s onwards" (2009, p. 33). A study of biographies, personal contacts, and personal exchanges with colleagues, in that case, can support a researcher with shards of evidence on the truth of their views.

> The discourse of Soviet science generally and, particularly, the discourse of social and human sciences from the 1930s onwards is most unusual and highly problematic for the Western reader, and one needs special skills and to possess a great wealth of background knowledge about the time, place and the cultural codes of the social organization of science in order to "decode" the message of this discourse, and without knowing these rules and discursive conventions one can hardly understand the development of Soviet human and behavioral sciences from the 1930s onwards.
> (Yasnitsky, 2009, p. 93)

While Miller, Etkind, and Rozhdestvensky made their conclusions on the basis of historical events and didn't go further into theoretical explorations of writings, produced by ex-followers of psychoanalysis after the 1930s, some Western scholars such as Joravsky and Calloway noted certain influences of psychoanalysis in Soviet psychology.[16] Before Stalin, Soviet psychology "was not at war with 'bourgeois' psychologists" (Joravsky, 1989, p. 233). After Stalin "Uznadze's disciples, the distinctive Georgian school of psychologists, have provided the chief centre for renewed interest in the Freudian unconscious" (p. 455, note 17).

Loren Graham pointed out that after the 1960s there were "a number of efforts in Soviet literature to show that Freud was by no means the first person to point to the importance of the subconscious realm" (Graham, 1988, note 94). This attempt was, no doubt, an attempt to relativize Freud, to make possible a turning of real attention to Freud without appearing to embrace Freudism after years of denying its legitimacy. "They have criticized the 'monopoly' of Freudism abroad ... But on the whole, they have been moving more and more toward a recognition of Freud" (p. 215). He then writes about Uznadze:

> And M.S. Lebedinskii, from the Institute of Psychiatry of the Academy of Medical Sciences, commented that presenting Uznadze as an alternative to Freud was an unsuccessful attempt, since a Freudian analyst would have no trouble accepting Uznadze's views and still remaining a loyal Freudian.
> (Graham, 1988, p. 216 and p. 471, note 100)

In the chapter dedicated to Luria we will see some evidence of the persecution that fell on him after 1930 that will explain why he "simply trained for a new profession" (Rozhdestvenskii, 2009).

As we have seen from the earlier discussion in this chapter, major components of the social practice of Soviet scientists, such as language, public behaviour, and styles of criticism were dramatically changed over the 1930s to 1950s. Added to them,

> the key instruments used to implement Stalinist Science were: state censorship; rituals of so-called "self-criticism" and politically motivated "public discussions"; the institutionalization of a new state-science bureaucracy; the creation of a new elitist ruling quasi-class of the Party *nomenklatura* (Voslensky, 1984); and dissemination and standardization of the rhetoric of Party 'newspeak' in scientific discourse. This resulted in a major paradox for Soviet science of the 1930s: the declaration of the exceptional role of science in society (which implies relative independence of science from other social institutions) and total state control over science (including the total dependence of Stalinist Science on its Party patrons). The situation was further aggravated by the growing international isolation of the Soviet Union from the mid-1930s onwards, which "dramatically contrasted with the international success and growing international recognition of Soviet science.
> (Yasnitsky, 2009, p. 43).

This created a designated territory for academics to practice within.

As Krementsov points out "by 1939, Soviet scientists understood perfectly well the principles of operation of the Stalinist science system and had learned to use that system to their own advantage" (Krementsov, 1996, p. 80). He also added that

> it is clear that from the end of the 1930s onwards only those individuals who thoroughly understood the real meaning of Soviet science policy and

the internal mechanics of decision-making in the country could make scientific careers in the Soviet Union.

(p. 75)

As we will see in the chapter dedicated to Bassin, his career path fits the description above. One of the early enthusiasts of psychoanalysis, he moved to Moscow from Kharkiv to join Luria and colleagues in their research and to develop his practice. Instead, he had to focus on electroencephalography, write a dissertation on the electrical activity of brain injuries and denounce his affiliation to Freud's ideas for a good 20 years. However, as soon as the possibility was open, he returned to discussing psychoanalysis, this time using the appropriate critical language, of course.

Now that the key presupposition for my work – the encrypted character of Soviet writings and negation as the core mechanism for it – has been introduced, it is time to return to the Freud Session. I will try to draw some facts from the contents of this session from its original source in Russian, published in the journal *Voprosy Filosofii* [Issues of Philosophy] (Bondarenko and Rabinovitch, 1959, pp. 164–170). If we do not take the criticism seriously and look only at the content of the speech of every presenter, the whole session will start looking like an exchange of the latest news in the field of Western psychoanalysis.

## The Freud Session, one more time

Semyon Sarkisov[17] made the opening statement. His started his speech by arguing that lately, in the West, Freudian ideas were more and more criticized. "The spread of Freudian ideas in the West lately caused the rise of the opposition towards his ideas from the progressive representatives of medicine, psychology and philosophy" (Bondarenko and Rabinovitch, 1959, p. 165). "All that *obliges*[18] Soviet scientists to take an active part in the ideological struggle against Freudism", he said.

This obligation to follow the Western path for a Soviet scientist sounds unusual, especially for 1958. I think it was precisely at this moment that academics had a chance to negotiate, once again, the boundaries and rules of ideological censorship. At the same time, by 1958, after a period of infiltration by ideology, and the establishment of State control over science, Soviet academics had begun using the discourse of the state to resist its authoritarian pressure. As Fitzpatrick notices, by the 1960s the older generation had already learned how to "speak Bolshevik",[19] whilst the younger were native speakers (Fitzpatrick, 2005, p. 25). But let's return to the session.

To continue his argument regarding Western scientists criticising Freud, Sarkisov quoted to the audience *American*[20] psychiatrist Joseph Wortis from his *Fragments of an Analysis with Freud,* who describes the method of psychoanalysis as totally unscientific. Another unusual turn, one may think: to quote an American author during the Soviet ideological session appears unexpected, at the least. Then Sarkisov told the audience that at the XX International Psychoanalytic Congress in Paris in 1957, a group of French analysts stood against a group of American analysts. At the time, he stated, there were a lot of contradictions within psychoanalytic society. He also mentioned several events, such as conferences and symposiums, like "Freud and Pavlov" in February 1957 in Freiburg, Germany. Thus, according to Sarkisov, Soviet scientists should join Western colleagues in the struggle against psychoanalytic ideas. For someone living behind the 'Iron Curtain', Sarkisov was rather well informed on what was happening with psychoanalytic movements in the West.

The next 'critic' presented was Bassin with a speech titled 'The Critical Analysis of Contemporary Freudism' where he presents the history of the development of psychoanalytic theory from drives to ego, super-ego, and censorship. He 'criticizes' Freud's attempt to apply his ideas on the origin of civilization, aggression, the death drive etc. Bassin mentions various schools within orthodox psychoanalysis, and competing schools of Ernst Kris, Rudolph Loewenstein and Heinz Hartmann. He discusses the development of Freud's ideas in the West and criticism of them. Bassin notices, however, that the influence of Freud abroad was still very present. One of the founders of cybernetics, Norbert Weiner, claims that basic principles of Freudism are deeply in tune with the ideas of recent physics. Psychoanalysis is widely used in art theory and literary studies and taken up by other disciplines outside psychology. Psychoanalysis still stays as an ideological basis for psychosomatic medicine, widespread in the United States. This little excerpt from the wide range of information on the development of psychoanalysis in the West, available from the speech of Bassin, can serve as a brief introduction to Freudian theory, rather than as a criticism.

Another thing that Bassin tries to do in his speech is to disengage the idea of the unconscious from psychoanalytic discourse. He affirms that study of the unconscious can be done without reliance on psychoanalysis, and some of Freud's ideas, of course, were studied already by Pavlov. As we will see in chapters specifically dedicated to Bassin and Uznadze, this trick was used by Bassin many times. The canon he developed is: denounce Freud, introduce in detail all his wrongdoings without suggesting anything else, mention the unconscious as a phenomena that requires attention, spend some time around Pavlov, say words like 'reflex', 'brain', 'neurophysiology' – and, *voila*, your text is ready.

So, the whole session at some point appears as an event, the aim of which is to create space for discussion and to inform a wide audience of the situation with psychoanalysis in the West. Psychiatrists Evgeny Popov and Oleg Kerbikov[21] in their speeches discussed the value of the concept of the Oedipal complex. They emphasized the Neo-Freudian movement, Horney and Sullivan, whose theory of the origin of neurosis focuses on Ego and unrealistic expectations, as well as frustrated wishes of all kinds of nature, not only sexual. And the ideological struggle aim was fading away when the director of the Institute of Psychiatry of the Ministry of Health of the USSR, Dmitry Fedotov,[22] read aloud one of the critical answers to his article "The Soviet View of Psychoanalysis", published in the *Monthly Review* in 1957. The point of his opponent, Norman Reider, is that it is "quite useless to answer to the old arguments of the Soviet authors, which are not a result of the objective scientific relation to psychoanalysis, but the expression of the official governmental point of view" (Bondarenko and Rabinovitch, 1959). To claim that the attitude towards psychoanalysis is set by the Soviet government and does not represent the position of scientists in the Soviet Union is impossible to imagine, even in such a form. And only with the knowledge that the whole event was a farce, would Fedotov say what he said to such a wide audience. Apart from his criticisms of Freud, in that article, Fedotov also noticed that "at the present time Soviet physicians, psychologists and physiologists read psychoanalytic works only for the purpose of keeping in touch with the scientific interests of our colleagues abroad. To meet this purpose of the Soviet scholars, our libraries subscribe to books and journals on psychoanalysis, along with other publications issued abroad".[23] So in 1957 psychoanalytic literature was, in fact, available for Soviet scholars.[24]

After Fedotov, N. I. Grashchenkov[25] and A. V. Snezhnevsky[26] in their presentations talked about "the origins of Freud's philosophical views" (Bondarenko and Rabinovitch, 1959, p. 168). They emphasized that Freud was never a materialist, even though he studied with "outstanding neurologists" Meynert, von Brücke and Charcot. In fact, he was an "idealist and mystic" who relied on Nietzsche and Schopenhauer in his work.

Other presenters, P. K. Anokhin and V. N. Miasishchev in their papers emphasized the need to engage with Freud's view critically with more deep exploration of it, rather than just superficially. Since Freud, the question of the unconscious is an important part of the study of a mind, and "no one yet seriously researched how accumulated residual impressions in the brain are used, how they affect the realm of consciousness and behaviour" (Bondarenko and Rabinovitch, 1959, p. 169), Anokhin argued.[27]

Further parts of the session were dedicated to the problem of dream interpretation and its critique by the group of researchers from Leningrad. However, their argument focuses on the fact that Freud's interpretation of dreams is not exclusive, and there is a variety of theories, for example, the Jungian approach to interpretation of dreams, and several more theories that are developed in West Germany. Of course, they point to Pavlovian physiology as being a suitable theory for further exploration of the dream-states.

The final bit of the Freud Session presents a critique of sociological ideas of Freud by Professor of Philosophy, Bondarenko. The main point he is making is that Freud's ideas are used by bourgeois sociologists to critique Marxism. He criticizes Franz Alexander for the 'colonial' application of psychoanalytic ideas and for labelling some nations as less developed and therefore promoting imperialist US views onto them. He discusses the application of the 'Oedipus complex' into thinking about the masses, and doubts Freud's suggestion that leaders are substitutes for the father figure[28] "for people, who experience longing for a father since their childhood". For him the main problem is that Freud reduced the masses to passive crowds and overlooked their ability as a class power.

In the conclusion of the session, it was noted that "the ideological struggle against Freudism caused great interest in the medical audience" (Bondarenko and Rabinovitch, 1959, p. 170).

\*

Many lines of this research come together when we analyse this event. It is, first, an event that can be read differently with hindsight. Reconstruction of the social context – an invisible counterpart for scientists, that accumulated language, ideology, and politics – allows us to see the Freud Session in a different light. Being done in different times and from inside and outside of the Soviet Union, historiographies of the Freud Session kept repeating each other. It is only with the introduction of the idea of resistance to the authoritarian discourse that the possibility of a different reading was opened. Attention to minor details in this perspective became of great importance and changed how the Freud Session is seen. The use of the psychoanalytic concept of negation allows us to deconstruct the meaning of the 'critique' and to suggest new ways of reading and understanding the Session.

A good example of the same kind of transformation from difficulty to revelation is a study of sciences of the child – pedology – by Andy Byford. He writes:

> However, what I soon came to realize was that to understand how and why a distinctive domain of knowledge formed around 'the child' at this historical juncture, it was not enough to study the institutional and epistemic structures of science itself. Rather, it was essential first to grasp the constitution of those social realms in which this emergent body of knowledge was acquiring meaning and pertinence precisely as "science".
> (Byford, 2020, ix).

Writing on pedology, Byford (2020) notices that the 'damnation' of it by the Communist Party "proved decisive in shaping the historiography of Russo-Soviet science to date" (p. 34) Why? His answer echoes Yasnitsky's argument about the reproduction of the Stalinist model of science in psychology. Byford finds out that "Crucial to 'forgetting' was also the fact that Soviet historiographies of science produced disciplinary histories as supporting pillars of particular disciplines' institutional existence *in the present* (the italics of the author)" (p. 35). That selection process impacted on how different scientific traditions and institutions were documented. Classification of 'good' and 'bad' school thoughts "served the function of disciplinary legitimation" (p. 35). As pedology was a '*failed* discipline', "the most that historians could and, in fact, did do was to affirm pedology's ultimate failure" (p. 35). For another failed discipline, psychoanalysis, that destiny was not too different.

Overall, this approach to historiography prompted me to reflect on a need for the distinction between two lines of interest for the current book: the history of psychoanalysis as a theory and the history of the psychoanalytic movement. By 'the history of the psychoanalytic movement' I mean the establishment of organizations before and after the revolution, the ban on psychoanalysis and interruption of psychoanalytic publishing and study, and an official return of psychoanalysis after the fall of the Soviet Union. That history is different from the history of psychoanalysis as a theory, psychoanalysis as a specific knowledge about the psyche, the theory of unconscious and the methodologies that are used to analyse culture and social phenomena.

It falls neither in the category of a 'Great Man' study, nor of the study of a 'bureaucratic transplant model' (Cameron and Forrester, 2017, p. 2) of psychoanalysis. Rather, it is a study of psychoanalytic ideas transferred through years of Soviet rule and transformations of these ideas under the circumstances of those years. One main focus and interest of my work is to distinguish between transformations done by the social and political reality and transformations that happened in minds of scholars who engaged with psychoanalysis and tried to apply it within the time they lived in. This is why I borrow the word 'vicissitudes' from the text of Freud's *Drives and their Vicissitudes* (1915b) to exactly highlight *the variety* of changes implemented in the destiny of psychoanalysis in Soviet Russia. Further chapters will be dedicated to the vicissitudes of psychoanalysis as a theory and an attempt to reconstruct its influence on the theories and practices invented by Soviet scientists. Nevertheless, this is not just a history of psychoanalysis in Soviet Russia or the history of the influence of psychoanalysis. This work attempts to bring back to the theory of mind original ideas of Soviet psychologists and physiologists.

Further chapters will attempt to what historians of psychoanalysis John Forrester and Laura Cameron conclude about work of Freud in Cambridge – basically, to acknowledge the intersection of physiology, neuropsychology and psychology with psychoanalytic ideas in the Soviet science, yet unacknowledged in the historiography:

> Undoubtedly the fact that these were all new disciplines in formation permitted these unpredictable influences to be felt. But what is equally striking is that the four disciplines [psychology, anthropology, English, philosophy] all, in the end, repudiated the influence of psychoanalysis.
> (Cameron and Forrester, 2017, p. 361)

As further chapters will show, in accordance with the course of the development of Soviet society, early followers of psychoanalysis and their pupils found the way to keep their scientific interests intact and formed a shield to protect from persecution for collaboration with anti-state ideas. This, however, caused several complications. Unlike in the cases of Jacques Lacan, Melanie Klein, and Wilfred Bion, who significantly transformed psychoanalytic theory and at the same time stayed within the Freudian tradition, not only theoretically developing psychoanalysis, but clinically practicing it, Luria and Vygotsky are rather perceived as authors outside of the psychoanalytic scene. In a pure sense these theories are not psychoanalytic ones, as they departed from the mainstream of the psychoanalytic debate. Nevertheless, alongside Zeigarnik, Bassin and Uznadze they bring a new contribution to that scene, as they are concerned with the main psychoanalytic issues: unconscious, thinking, language, and the origin of neuroses and psychoses. Moreover, they are not only concerned with the mind, but consider the individual as a whole: a body with a mind. At the same time, they cannot be seen as fully independent from psychoanalytic discourse, because ignoring their psychoanalytic roots distorts the meaning of theoretical and clinical findings of these theories. That leads to oversimplification, and as post-Soviet history has shown, an effective abandonment of Soviet theories as outdated or portrayal of them as isolationist and departed from psychoanalysis.

## Notes

1 For an account on the relationship between the psychoanalytic movement and the prohibition of pedology see Byford, 2020.
2 We can see already that most of these histories were written around 20 years ago. Since then not much has been produced on this topic and, perhaps, this is another question to answer – why?
3 Pedology (Greek παιδός – a child + λόγος – a science) – is a neologism used by Soviet practitioners to refer to a branch of pedagogy that aimed to unite medical, psychological, physiological knowledge and to form a science of child development.
4 Indeed, further development of mental health care in Soviet Union has led to the appearance of multiple forms of schizophrenia and domination of that diagnosis. That shift and its reasons will be discussed in detail in the following chapter.
5 More about the role of Miasishchev in lobbying inclusion of psychology in the curriculum for doctors and psychiatrists and re-establish the Institute of Psychology in 1948, is in Benjamin Zajicek's work "Scientific Psychiatry in Stalin's Soviet Union: the Politics of Modern Medicine and the Struggle to Define 'Pavlovian' Psychiatry, 1939–1953" (PhD thesis, University of Chicago, 2009).
6 Rosental published on Dostoevsky novellas in 1920 while Freud's study on Dostoevsky appeared only in 1927.
7 Relations of Soviet State with sexuality is another important topic some scholars engaged with in a quite detailed way in works of Keti Chukhrov (2020) and Aaron Shuster (2016).
8 Much like *Psychosocial Studies* today.
9 For institutional history, the establishment of the IPA training model in Russia and difficulties of the post-Soviet psychoanalytic institutions see Kadyrov, 2005; Kadyrov, 2013.
10 As we will see in the chapter dedicated to the presence of Freud in the Soviet press, some of Freud's ideas were a sort of a common knowledge for the public.
11 The atmosphere of this form of communal living was represented, for example, by the movie *Khrustalyov, mashinu!* (*Khrustalyov, My Car!*) (1998) by Alexei German, a Soviet and Russian director.

Michael Cole in his memoires on the meeting with Luria mentions poor conditions in which Luria's family had to exist.

12 See Yasnitsky, 2015.
13 For a detailed outline of different schools of psychology and their destiny after 1930s see Bogdanchikov, 2020.
14 "In the depth of his heart he knew he was dying, but not only was he not accustomed to the thought, he simply did not and could not grasp it".

The syllogism he had learnt from Kiesewetter's Logic: "Caius is a man, men are mortal, therefore Caius is mortal", had always seemed to him correct as applied to Caius, but certainly not as applied to himself. That Caius – man in the abstract – was mortal, was perfectly correct, but he was not Caius, not an abstract man, but a creature quite, quite separate from all others". Leo Tolstoy, *The death of Ivan Ilych* (1886).

15 Fitzpatrick notices in *Tear Off the Masks!* (2005), that the need to conceal something about their life was permanent for citizens of the USSR, however, depending on the decade the focus on what exactly had to be kept private was on different questions. If in the 1920s it was the pre-Revolutionary past, in the 1930s the accusation shifted to the spy and the enemy of the state. Connections with foreigners was under the attention of authorities especially during the war. Luria, Zeigarnik, Uznadze studied abroad and had to hide their international connections. Luria was persecuted for over ten years for his early engagement with psychoanalysis and his international network. In the late 1940s and early 1950s anti-Semitic campaigns brought into focus his Jewish origin. Bassin, Luria, Vygotsky and Zeigarnik were Jews and apart from Vygotsky who died before it, suffered from the anti-Semitic campaign.
16 Joravsky (1989), for example, writes about Vygotsky and Luria *Etiudy* "Vygotsky and Luria borrowed heavily and quite respectfully from such Western authorities as Piaget and Freud" (p. 233). Calloway (1992), "Despite the criticism of psychoanalysis, Soviet psychiatrists are less dismissive of psychoanalysis than is commonly thought" (p. 110).
17 Sarkisov was neurophysiologist and held the position of the director of the Moscow Brain Institute for 40 years. He was a member of the Academy of Sciences. His activity on the front of Soviet psychiatry, and especially discussions about the use of lobotomy, is discussed in detail by Benjamin Zajicek (2009). From Zajicek's research it is clear also, that Sarkisov was experienced in 'criticism' and chairing scientific sessions. In archives on Bassin at GARF, we find documents indicating that a year before the Freud Session, in 1957, Sarkisov chaired the dissertation defence of Bassin, and in his concluding speech stated that "Unfortunately, at the last session of the Academy of Medical Sciences there were comments about the fact that we are not sufficiently opposed to these ideological concepts that are alien to us. I want to express my full satisfaction that Bassin is one of the scientists who opposes these perversions, and not only in this current work, but we know of his reasonable speeches in the Journal of Higher Nervous Activity against these ideological perversions. *This is one of the indicators of the maturity of a Soviet scientist*" (the translation and emphasis is mine) (GARF, f.P-9506, o.16, d.213, p. 219). It could be that Bassin was protected by the reputation of Sarkisov and his passion for criticism and used him as a solid cover.
18 The emphasis is mine.
19 'To speak Bolshevik' is a phrase used by historian Stephen Kotkin in his work *Magnetic Mountain* (1995). It describes the adoption of the language of the State by its citizens in order to achieve their goals. This phenomenon is described by Fitzpatrick and Krylova, whose critique is more related to the question of identity, which is, as they suggest, more complex than citizens adopting Soviet values or opposing them.

20 The emphasis is mine.
21 It is important to notice that despite the criticism, whether genuine or not, the Handbook of Psychiatry authored by a collective including Popov, Kerbikov and Snezhnevsky mentions psychoanalysis in the chapter dedicated to the Western Psychiatry of the 19$^{th}$–20$^{th}$ Century. Kerbikov O.V, Korkina M.V, Nadzharov R. A., Snezhnevsky A.V. Psikhiatriia. Uchebnik. M: Meditsina 1968, pp. 24–25 [Psychiatry. Handbook. Moscow, Medicine].
22 The establishment of Fedotov's psychiatric career is presented in detail in Benjamin Zajicek's work (2009). Curiously, Zajicek noticed that his promotion by officials was "particularly striking, because Fedotov's success was built on blatant violations of the law" (p. 94).
23 Published in appendix of Baran, Paul A. (1960) *Marxism and Psychoanalysis*. (Monthly review pamphlet series). Monthly Review Press; First Edition, pp. 55–56.
24 Twenty years later, in 1978 Fedotov also took part in Volume II of the materials for the Congress on Unconscious in Tbilisi, which happened a year later, in 1979. In his article titled 'On the Problem of the Unconscious in Psychiatry' he discusses the nature of such states as depersonalization, psychic automatism, and suicide as a representation of unconscious intentions. Fedotov had worked on the problem of suicide since 1970 and was the founder of the Soviet suicidology. He is an author of *A Feature Story of the History of Domestic Psychiatry* first published in 1957 and continuously republished up until 2017.
25 The career and his way to the 'top administrators' for Grashchenkov is presented in detail in Zajicek's research (2009, p. 255). Grashchenkov was the one who appointed Luria to be in charge of the hospital in Kisegach during the war, and "after the war Grashchenkov continued to support Luria and his research, and together they published a series of papers in which they proposed a theory of consciousness based on what they referred to as "functional systems". These functional systems, they argued, were made possible by the chemical transmission of nerve impulses: the synapse, not the reflex, was the basic constitutive unit of the mind" (p. 262). In this article, notes Zajicek, what was remarkable was the fact that "they did not cite Lenin's theory of "reflection" *at all*, nor did they mention Ivan Pavlov, two omissions that were practically unheard of in a paper that dealt with how the brain formed a dynamic response to the world around it" (p. 273) That absence of citations is, indeed, striking and allows us to suggest that Grachenkov, perhaps, was not a blind ideological functionary.
26 A father of 'sluggish schizophrenia' and prominent figure of the psychiatric abuse, Snezhnevsky by the 1958 was quite a powerful figure in Soviet psychiatry, so that explains his presence in the session. His career is discussed in Zajicek (2009, p. 104). From his story there is no evidence of masquerade, but the opposite – Snezhnevsky seem to have felt quite comfortable with the regime.
27 Anokhin's scientific interests were concerned with conscious and unconscious activity. The school of Anokhin and his theory of functional systems as opposed to the reflex had a great influence on Luria. The notion of "satisfactory scheme" or "feedback", perhaps, is the most important of Anokhin's discoveries, achieved 12 years before the origin of cybernetics and anticipating a lot of its postulates.
28 This is especially curious detail, as in 1958 the whole nation was still mourning a great Father Stalin.

Chapter 2

# Freud in the public discourse

This chapter will provide a context of three more dimensions of the public discourse that closely related to the vicissitudes of psychoanalysis. These are: the new policy towards sexuality; representation of Freud and psychoanalysis in the public press; and clinical directions of psychotherapy in general.

As we've seen in the previous chapter, a huge shift in society after the establishment of the USSR was not only applied to economic and political changes. Reconstruction in science, scientific institutes, and education transformed what should be considered knowledge. Changes in social institutions led to the transformation of morals and social rules, which impacted individuals' consciousness and perception. These changes are intimately linked with the 'disappearance' of sex in the USSR, or rather the work of negation applied to sex. This was effected in the establishment of the new libidinal economy of the Soviet individual and made an invisible contribution to the perception and circulation of psychoanalysis in the public discourse.

In the first decade after the 1917 Revolution a lot of discussion on the role of sexuality in mental functioning and the genesis of neuroses circulated in texts of Soviet authors. For example, Luria in 'Psychoanalysis of the Costume' [Psikhoanaliz Kostiuma] (1922) puts sexuality and expression of drives at the core of the motivation for creation of clothes. Sabina Spielrein in her review 'Russian Literature on Psychoanalysis' for the Beihefte der IZP (1921), where she names most of early followers of the psychoanalytic movement, notices how heated were discussions about the role of sexuality in development of neuroses among clinicians at that time (Ovcharenko, 2006). Very soon, however, and not without the effort of Zalkind, who at first found it important to pay attention to Freud's theory of sexual drives (1924), but changed his argument dramatically (in his Twelve Statements, also in 1924) into attack, words like 'pansexualism' became attached to Freud's name. This happened not for theoretical reasons, but in tune with political and social changes that I will briefly introduce further. They also constituted a new public discourse around sexuality, perfectly illustrated by the following famous episode from the end of the time of the Soviet rule. It will serve as the starting point for our thinking.

DOI: 10.4324/9781003527268-3
This chapter has been made available under a CC-BY-ND 4.0 license.

In 1986, while hosting a live TV Bridge between Leningrad and Boston, an American woman raised the topic of sex. She said that Americans had a lot of sex on TV and in commercials and asked whether Soviets have the same problem. The Soviet woman's response became legendary. She said: "We have no sex in the USSR and we are very much against it".[1] Barely anyone remembers the question anymore, or the context of the conversation, but the phrase stuck in history as a description of the paradox: there was no sex in the USSR, but somehow new citizens were getting born. 'No sex' is a classic example of the work of the negation that was built through the Soviet years.

Immediately after the Revolution in 1917, there was a shift from the puritan Tsarist Russian policy towards a huge Soviet liberation. That included changes in both social attitudes and official government policy. Since the Revolution aimed to liberate people from the suppression of the monarchy and church, a new Soviet person should not in any way be like the old regime person. Changes in policy towards sex and sexuality were mainly concerned with the family and reproductive regulations. The Family Code in 1918 abolished old laws regarding marriage, divorce, and abortions. It introduced women's equality[2]; homosexuality was removed from the criminal code; the procedure of marriage and divorce shifted from the church to civil authorities. Overall, enlightenment and education went hand in hand with freedom from the patriarchal family. However, the question of sex would immediately bring up the question of raising children (Goldman, 1993, p. 8), since reliable contraception was mainly abortion. Some of the social promises, like communal dining rooms (*stolovaia*) and kindergartens, were supposed to help with practicalities and free women from household labour and the upbringing of children, so they could use their time to work and to think, and supposedly free sex from the 'consequences' of additional burden. Thus, sexual issues were social from the very beginning.

On the level of reality, liberation brought additional troubles to citizens, whose lives became even more chaotic with these freedoms. An idealistic expectation that relations between sexes were going to be regulated by free will and mutual attraction led to a rise in divorces, criminal abortions, single motherhood, abandoned children, and prostitution. While it was not due to freedom itself, but rather because of the devastation of the economy, Civil War, and ideological struggle, which was not possible to stabilize in a short period of time, it was decided that something should be done with freedoms instead. By the 1930s, laws became even stricter than in the Tsarist regime (Goldman, 1993). Citizens would not anymore have to spend their time troubled with sexual relationships and their consequences, their energy had to be saved for work. Under Stalin a family, and not an individual, became again the 'cell of the society'.

> Couching the new policies in a populist appeal for social order, the Party abandoned its earlier vision of social relations in favour of a new reliance

on mass repression. The 'withering-away' doctrine, once central to the socialist understanding of the family, law, and the state, was anathemized.

(Goldman, 1993, p. 296–297)

Moreover, the duty of raising children was returned to women, who now had to hold the 'double burden' of work and household. Bohemian circles had vanished too: "art during Stalin's time, and Soviet art for years after Stalin's death, was also extremely puritanical and sexually repressive" (Suny, 2011, p. 296).

That shift was reflected also in attitudes toward homosexuality. After being decriminalized in the first years of the Revolution, by the 1930s

> Family life became the subject of perspective scrutiny, where before Bolshevik leaders had said little about the internal dynamics and psychology of the husband- wife relationship. *Pravda* condemned 'so-called "free love" and all disorderly sex life' as unquestionably bourgeois and against Soviet morality and pointed out the dominant pattern of family relations among the 'elite of our country [who] are as a rule also excellent family men who dearly love their children'.
>
> (Healey, 2001, p. 198)

Any sexual activity that was not aimed at reproduction was proclaimed a disorder. In 1935, psychiatrist E.A. Popov radically deconstructed "homosexuality" as a category of mental illness. "The state abruptly shifted the nexus of medico-legal supervision of same-sex love to practitioners of forensic medicine and gynaecology, disciplines undergoing significant restructuring as a result of the Five-Year Plans" (Healey, 2001, p. 193).

Among these shifts in the family codes, that presumably aimed to regulate social problems like divorce, prostitution, growing numbers of children without parents – *besprizorniki*, etc. – there was also negotiation over how much individual freedom, including sexual freedom, should be allowed without posing a danger to the regime. It was, of course, not only the problem of taking care of children, but it was also a question of libidinal investments.

The tension was formulated by Aaron Shuster in his preface to Andrei Platonov's Anti-Sexus:

> If part of the twentieth century's revolutionary program to create a radically new social relation and a New Man was the liberation of sexuality, this aspiration was marked by a fundamental ambiguity: Is it sexuality that is to be liberated, delivered from moral prejudices and legal prohibitions, so that the drives are allowed a more open and fluid expression, or is humanity to be liberated from sexuality, finally freed from its obscure dependencies and tyrannical constraints?
>
> (Shuster, 2016. p. 22)

Aron Zalkind, an early enthusiast and enthusiastic critic of psychoanalysis, presented his view on liberation from sexuality in *The Revolution and Young People* (1924), where he put forward his famous 'Twelve sexual precepts of the revolutionary proletariat' in which he formulates in a near-biblical way, the restrictions of sexuality. This included the prohibition of early sexual life; a requirement that sexual life begin only after marriage; a proposal for rare sexual intercourses even for married couples, etc. Some restrictions appear to be prohibiting pleasure at large. The progeny must be borne in mind on each occasion of the sexual act. Sexual choice should be made on the basis of class and revolutionary expediency. There must not be the use of the weaponry of sexual conquest – coquetry, flirtation, courtship. These carry a class function, not a personal one. Class virtues, not purely physiological allurements, must be victorious. There must be no jealousy. There must be no sexual perversion.[3]

These regulations around sex, however, point to the fact that sexuality was not really excluded from Soviet life. Actually, it was constantly present there, but in the negated form. 'Sex did not exist', 'sex should not be practiced outside the marriage', 'a sexual act must not be frequently repeated' – all these formulations are reminders of the existence of a sexual drive and the attempt to deny it. Besides, sex was often a topic of discussion in the main political newspaper, *Pravda*, a topic for short stories and novels written by Soviet authors, and the largest attendance in the regular communal meetings was achieved when the topic for discussion touched on sex and sexuality. As Eric Naiman concludes: "We can read Soviet discourse on sexuality in 1926 and 1927 as precisely … a process in which discussion was first eroticised so that it could ultimately be more effectively politicised" (Naiman, 1997, p. 101).

The discontent of psychoanalysis in these circumstances might appear as self-evident, as it was constantly bringing the sexual into consciousness and thus into the possession of the individual. With psychoanalysis the 'trick' of negation did not work. While the official story was that critics accused Freud of 'pansexuality' and diminishing the complexity of the individual to the animalistic level, I think it was rather the competition for owning drives, that now had to belong to the State, that caused the attack. How could it be allowed for psychoanalysis to deal with libidinal drives if they were now appropriated by the State?

A curious episode of the return of sex occurred during The Symposium on The Unconscious in Tbilisi in 1979. At the roundtable with French psychoanalysts, who used words very unusual for Soviet ears like 'phallus' and 'sexuality', the chair of the session, a Soviet professor of psychology, was blushing. At some point she started to denounce Freud. She listed the usual criticisms, like bourgeoise etc, and especially that he reduced everything to sexuality and this is not right, because "in the mind we have not only sexual presentations, but also everyday life, scientific, legal, philosophical and other sexual presentations". Of course, that was a Freudian slip that was immediately noticed by the audience, which burst into laughter and applause (Mazin, 2019, pp. 106–107).

If, in academia, regulations were implemented by appointed Party functionaries, the masses got their directions from newspapers, owned and regulated by the state. The same mechanisms, however, were in place in the public press, which became a source of criticism and information about Freud and psychoanalysis.

## Freud and psychoanalysis in the Soviet Press 1920–1980

> Binary accounts of socialism that describe it in terms of truth and falsity or official knowledge and unofficial knowledge fail to recognize precisely this performative dimension of authoritative language, reducing it instead to the constative dimension. Since authoritative discourse did not provide an accurate constative description of reality and since no competing description of reality was widely available, one could conclude that the late Soviet world became a kind of 'postmodern' universe where grounding in the real world was no longer possible, and where reality became reduced to discursive simulacra.
> (Yurchak, 2005, p. 75).

This section continues to explore the effects of the 'language affair' and will add some details from the Soviet archive of the contemporary press to represent the reception of psychoanalysis outside academia during 1900–1980. Since newspapers and journals constituted an important channel for authoritative discourse and adopted the language of the official ideology, they've constructed a 'public picture' of psychoanalysis. At the same time, as we will see, we can find elements of the same discrete techniques and use of the official language to keep the conversation about psychoanalysis alive. The basis for the analysis of the press that I attempt in this part was provided by all the above-mentioned studies of different aspects of Soviet life. As we have seen, all of them captured the same phenomena, although describing it in different terms, which I suggest understanding through the notions of splitting and negation. Splitting was an important part of everyday life, observed in practices related to politics and ideology, and present in the functioning of the economic system. Negation was a mechanism that helped to keep elements of life – like sex, and prohibited sciences like psychoanalysis – present in the discourse.

In fact, it was difficult to capture views on psychoanalysis between 1930 and 1980, because it was neither present nor absent. It was not 'not present'. But, as we know, double negation does not equal affirmation and it only points to the presence of the phenomena, without registering it in its reality. That's why we are getting close to the notion of the postmodernist 'discursive simulacra'. As Yurchack argues, "in fact, precisely because authoritative language was hegemonic, unavoidable, and hypernormalized, it was no longer read by its audiences literally, at the level of constative meanings" (2005, p. 76). To illustrate this, he brings the example of two girls using the 'District Party Committee [*raikom*] meeting' as an excuse to miss university seminars for visiting an exhibition or cafe. While their professors or bosses knew it was not *raikom* meetings these girls were going to attend, they would be unlikely to say no as the reason was described in the authoritative symbols – *raikom* (pp. 120–121). "In short, they were able to deterritorialize time, space, relations, and meanings of the socialist system by drawing on the system's principles" (p. 121).

By delving into the pages of newspapers, I am hoping to show how Freud's name became 'not present' and 'not known', but widely and repeatedly circulated. The public press was monitored by Party authorities, so the system of censorship acting during that time was applied to the newspapers in the same way as to scientific publications. So, from newspapers and journals we also get a better understanding of the years of the 'ban' on psychoanalysis in academia in the 1930s and the return of interest in the unconscious after 'the Thaw' in the 1960s. We will see, nevertheless, that Freud's name never disappeared from public discourse, and the word 'psychoanalysis' infiltrated everyday language.

My research was conducted through the digitalized archive of the Soviet Press via the East View database among 7,699 periodicals between 1900 and 1981. Primary keywords results were for 'psychoanalysis'[4] – 212 matches, for 'Freud' – 457 matches and 'Freudism' – 130 matches. Most of them appeared in the newspapers *Pravda*,[5] *Izvestiia*,[6] *Nedelia, Literaturnaia Gazeta*,[7] *Sovetskaia kul'tura*[8] and the journals *Krokodil*[9] and *Ogonek*.[10]

## Where Freud becomes 'not legitimate'

Although my research primarily focused on the years 1930–1980 this section will look at the antecedent years to trace changes in the attitude to Freud more fully. Specifically, I am interested in the transition from a welcoming tone to a hostile attitude towards him. As we have seen from the discussion on the existing narrative about the 'ban' of psychoanalysis, it is still uncertain when exactly this shift happened and why. There was no decree prohibiting psychoanalysis, although its 'disappearance' is attributed in the literature to the 1930s with different versions of why it happened. Just to remind the reader, as we saw in the Chapter 1, that it was the gradual rise of repressions in the mid-1930s (Angelini, 2008), a loss of interest in psychoanalysis due to the lack of clinical effectiveness (Rozhdestvenskii, 2009), or a mixture of political and cultural reasons, due to the attack from Soviet Marxists (Etkind, 1997; Miller, 1998; Hristeva and Bennett, 2018). Here I present some additional evidence from newspapers of the mid-1920s where we will see the attack on psychoanalysis from the main ideologists of Marxism and show that by the 1930s the official ideology was already in opposition to psychoanalysis.

The first appearance of psychoanalysis in the public press was relatively late, compared to academic activity around psychoanalysis. In 1922, *Izvestiia* (No. 225) announced the establishment of the Russian Psychoanalytic Society. The same year *Pravda* (1922, No. 258) announced the publication of Freud's

Introductory Lectures on Psychoanalysis. In 1923 in an article about events in Poland, the author makes a passing comment that Freud's theory has a prosperous future (*Pravda*, 1923, No. 165). Next year only two mentions of psychoanalysis came out without criticism: the announcement of the book On Psychoanalysis of the Children's Years by a collective of authors Karl Abraham, Ernest Jones, Carl Yung, Victor Tausk et al, (*Pravda*, 1924, No. 169) and that Vygotsky will present his paper at the meeting of the Russian Psychoanalytic Society (*Izvestiia*, 1924, No. 278).

Hristeva and Bennett (2018) suggest that it was 1924 when the discussion about the compatibility of Freud with Marxism started. In that year the journal *Pod Znamenem Marxisma* (Under the Banner of Marxism) No. 8–9 August-September published a critical paper 'Freudism and Marxism' by Jurinetz. Indeed, we find in this a footnote under the title saying, "The editors consider one of the immediate tasks of Marxist philosophy to criticize Freud and Freudism from the point of view of dialectical materialism" (Jurinetz, 1924, p. 51). The response in newspapers did not take long. Already in October of that year, *Pravda* (1924, No. 225) published a review by S. Volodin on Ivan Ermakov's book *Essays on the Oeuvre of Gogol*. The opening line of this review stated: "Ermakov – is a supporter of Freud". The tone of the review was very critical, and the author concluded that Ermakov's analysis illustrates how the Freudian method is useless in understanding social phenomena. Following the discussion opened by *Pod Znamenem Marxisma*, a debate on the question of Freudism and Marxism was held in the Moscow Publishing House in February 1925. The publication about it appeared in *Pravda* (1925, No. 49); Alexander Luria is mentioned there as one of the contributors.

Throughout 1925 the amount of criticism towards Freud in *Pravda* and *Izvestiia* grew, as review after review condemned Freudism. After the publication of *Beyond the Pleasure Principle* (3000 copies, published by the private publishing house of Nikolay Stolliar in Russian the same year) Freud was presented as a completely reactionary author (*Pravda*, 1925, No. 146). Freud was incompatible with Marxism (*Izvestiia*, 1925, No. 192), Freud was against physiology, anatomy, he was a member of the Masonic lodge, he was a mystic. The review said there is no science in psychoanalysis, it is a totally bourgeois idealistic theory (*Izvestiia*, 1925, No. 218). That did not stop the practice immediately, for example, the same year *Izvestiia* (No. 270) published the call from the Commissariat for Health [*Narodnyi Kommisariat Zdravookhraneniia*] advertising positions in the State Neuro-Psychiatric Dispensary (day clinic), and among them is a position of psychoanalyst. This corresponds with the evidence that psychoanalysis was practised by doctors sporadically even during WWII.[11]

After 1925, targeted attacks on psychologists with even a distant connection to Freud started to appear in book reviews columns in *Pravda* and *Izvestiia*. Kornilov was attacked for criticising reflexology and experimental psychology and using the term unconscious. "Apparently, Kornilov is Freud's follower", concludes the reviewer (*Izvestiia*, 1925, No. 273). In the same vein, Zalkind was attacked by the reviewer for similarities with Freud's ideas in his book A Sexual Question in Circumstances of the Soviet Society. "Not to mention, – adds the reviewer – that Zalkind's denunciation of Freud is superficial. In the core he is a true Freudist!" (*Pravda*, 1926, No. 123). Ivan Ermakov was put in danger for his introduction to Freud's book published in 1925 under the title *On Children's Neuroses*. The reviewer found 'very suspicious' that Ermakov "admires Freud and says nothing about the reactionary character of his theory" (*Pravda*, 1926, No. 136).

In 1926, several more reviews appeared strongly criticizing Freud's books and Freudism. A regular book review column in *Pravda* (No. 65) gives us a good summary of the main failures of psychoanalysis. There are reactionary philosophical elements in it, idealism, a theory of life as an aspiration to death, to nirvana etc. (presented in texts *Beyond the Pleasure Principle, The Ego and The Id*) as well as Oedipus complex and sublimation. After the publication of *The Psychology of the Dream*, this list was completed with mysticism and sexualism (*Pravda*, 1926, No. 149). It looks like by the end of 1926, the official position towards Freud had already been formulated, and in the following years reviewers no longer spent time arguing why Freud was wrong, referring to previous issues of *Pravda*, where 'this topic was already widely discussed'.

In 1927 Freud's name disappeared from book reviews, and the campaign against Freudism had been completed. The gradual dissolution of the psychoanalytic movement was inevitable and the main enthusiasts of it had to suspend their activities. This was the year when Alexander Luria resigned from the position of secretary in the Russian Psychoanalytic Society. Despite it being suggested that Luria left due to his growing interest in Gestalt psychology (Hames, 2002) or because psychoanalysis was never his primary interest (Proctor, 2020), the version that Luria predicted further political implications of his relations with psychoanalysis (Hristeva and Bennett, 2018) has support from the Soviet press where we see clearly the campaign against Freud and targeted criticism against his followers between 1924–1927.[12]

Thus, we see, how between 1924 and 1927 the official vocabulary of the critique of psychoanalysis had been formed. A template included: idealist, reactionary, bourgeois, mystical, pansexual, and was not changed in further years, so everyone willing to compose a text with Freud's name mentioned in it could just pick up one or several words from this template. Although it does not mean that there was a thoughtful critical attitude toward Freud or psychoanalysis, the repetition of the template over time served the purpose of the discursive simulacra that underpinned authoritative discourse by multiplying and repeating it. In the same way, the names of Marx, Engels and Lenin served as the opening line for any scientific text. This is also a powerful illustration of how newspapers were able to form public opinion and influence processes in science and in society.

From 1930, the debate around psychoanalysis, Freud and Freudism moved predominantly to pages of the newspapers *Literaturnaia gazeta* and *Sovetskoe iskusstvo*, occasionally appeared in the journal *Ogonek* and the newspapers *Pravda, Izvestiia* and *Nedelia*, and was more often mentioned in the journal *Krokodil*. Most of the discussion was situated in the field of art and touched on the use of psychoanalytic theory in literature, theatre, painting, and cinema.

Depending on the decade, the reason why psychoanalysis is wrong slightly varied, compared to the template used in *Pravda* and *Izvestiia*. In the 1930s, reviewers of foreign literature discuss the emergence of a new type of hero, a weak person, preoccupied with psychoanalysis of his internal reality and therefore distracted from participation in social processes. In contrast, "unconscious drives and motives are no longer important for the new Soviet man, who is preoccupied with the building of society rather than wasting time on reflecting on his internal conflicts" (*Literaturnaia gazeta*, 1930, No. 39). In that regard, Freud was put in line with Dostoevsky, who is known for "excessive psychologising, darkness and 'corrosive psychoanalysis'" (*Sovetskoe iskusstvo*, 1931, No. 7). Psychoanalysis was linked to the "abstraction, departed from life and analysing is equated to the preparation of the corpse" (*Literaturnaia gazeta*, 1932, No. 54).

At the peak of Stalin's repressions, 1936–1938, there was no word about psychoanalysis, even in the form of criticism. Several papers mentioned Freud as an author who contributed to the reactionary ideology in the literature and served to create anti-Leninist theory and Trotskyism (*Literaturnaia gazeta*, 1937, No. 30, No. 34). Up to 1948 Freud was rarely mentioned and when he was it was as an author who "abolished social and praised individualistic, animalistic, primitive motives of the human" (*Pravda*, 1947, No. 167).

These 'primitive, animalistic' motives of the Freudian human persisted in the centre of the critique of Hollywood productions and American theatre, because it was held that Freud could justify murders and sexual perversions of any kind. Reviews that appeared in the *Literaturnaia gazeta* and *Sovetskoe iskusstvo* through the 1950s and 1960s mostly showed the 'decomposition' and 'decay' of western culture, lost in psychoanalysis. In some reviews dedicated to new Alfred Hitchcock movies or Federico Fellini, in reports from Cannes festival, or discussion of the new view on Shakespeare in New York or Rome theatre, it was no longer clear whether the critique of psychoanalysis was genuine. Freud was not political or dangerous to the communist society, and only an echo of the struggle against Freudism from the 1930s passed from year to year. In the same vein as Freud's Session of 1958, writers for these newspapers were eager to fight against decaying western culture, but first they studied it, read it, watched its movies, and visited its cultural events.

In the 1970s, hardly any criticism of Freud can be found in the press, more a slight disagreement or simple mention without any judgement. He is the source of inspiration to Salvador Dali, to Alfred Hitchcock, to Bernardo Bertolucci. Tolstoy and Dostoevsky are rehabilitated, too, and together with Freud they represent a cohort of thinkers who deeply understood human nature. A lot of characters in translated literature confess that they undergo psychoanalytic treatment.

Overall, reading Soviet newspapers and journals it was striking to see how Freud's name truly managed to become common knowledge and infiltrated everyday language. Despite the repression of his ideas, Freud's name remained in the circulation and hence was available for the public.

## Where Freud's name circulates in public discourse

There are multiple examples of psychoanalytic ideas and thoughtful reference to Freud in articles and published novels not aiming to criticize psychoanalysis or denounce Freudism. In these examples the word 'psychoanalysis' was used as a common noun, and depending on the year it held negative or neutral connotations. Freud's name was called on when someone needed more understanding of the situation, or if the sexual meaning of someone's interaction had to be revealed, and in a joking manner (he looked at her in a 'Freudian' way). For instance, Nikolai Bukharin (*Pravda*, 1925, No. 260) referred to Freud as common knowledge in his attack on Ustryalov: "because [Nikolay] Ustryalov obviously finds narcissistic (according to Freud) pleasure in admiring his own style".

An interesting advertisement offering a course on oratory appeared in every issue of *Pravda, Izvestiia* and *Krokodil* for two years, 1927 and 1928. The course was titled "The mastery of arguing and joking" and was supposedly based on the writings of Prof Freud and Prof Gerling (whose identity I could not trace). The organizer asked to send pre-payment to Penza to receive materials for the course. The organizer must have relied on the common knowledge of Freud's ideas and attractiveness of his name to put money for two years of advertising in the major newspapers of the country.

The satirical journal *Krokodil* in 1928 (No. 14) came up with Soviet dream interpretations. Constructed as a typical book of interpretations of dreams, nevertheless, it gave credit to Freud's method. The list of symbols was clever and witty. The author of the article in *Ogonek* (1933, No. 23) about German nationalists shows familiarity with Freud's work *Totem and Taboo*, where "he writes about people from the islands in the Pacific ocean, who eat their ancestors to become like them". Another piece in *Krokodil* in 1933 (No. 15) brought an example of Freud as the resource of understanding in the situation. It is a short story about a man, who suddenly started thinking and even, became thoughtful about his work. That was such unusual behaviour, so his colleagues suspected: something must be wrong! "Someone suggested that he is in unrequited love and therefore started to switch to the social work – this called by Freud a sublimation". Apart from capturing beautifully someone not quite enthusiastic about work at the beginning of the Second Five Year Plan, an author here quite accurately applies the idea of sublimation.

In the same vein, Freud is mentioned in a short satirical story about a boy who couldn't master the Russian language at school and got bad marks and lots of corrections from his teacher. The confused parents didn't know why and couldn't understand their son's trouble with the language. At the point of desperation, as the author puts it, they were ready to 'call Freud' to help! Luckily, the problem solved itself another way – it turned out, that the teacher was illiterate (*Izvestiia*, 1934, No. 97). Or, in news about the Japanese decision to exit the Washington Naval Treaty in 1934 (*Izvestiia*, No. 305) the author concluded: "Because Japanese don't read Freud, they don't know about the existence of the inferiority complex".

Sources of knowledge about Freud and psychoanalysis spread through unpredictable channels. From the diary of a crew member on SS Chelyuskin, Michail Markov, we discover that on 28 January 1933,

> Otto Shmidt [a polar explorer, the head of the expedition and a member of the Russian Psychoanalytic Society] read a lecture about Freud to the crew. Despite the late hour the room was full, and everyone listened eagerly and after it was finished regretted it was over so quickly.
> (*Pravda*, 1934, No. 147)

That was not the only example of the informal circulation of Freud. His name kept recurring on pages of the press in further years. For example, in *Krokodil* (1936, No. 5) one of the army 'experts' when analysing his motives, says: "Perhaps, according to Freud's theory, my unconscious...". Or in a dramatic story, which took place in the provincial town Kostroma (*Izvestiia*, 1937, No. 152): a trial started against a young man who was accused because a girl had fallen in love with him and he didn't reciprocate, so that damaged her life. Freud's concept of obsessive thoughts was applied by his advocate to explain the girl's state and therefore proved the innocence of that young man. Some more news of Freud's use in the crime scene we find in *Izvestiia* (1940, No. 232): the defender of a victim highlighted that offenders tried to use psychoanalysis to attribute the guilt to the woman they had attempted to kill.

Decades later, the interest in Freud persisted among the young generation. In 1963 *Literaturnaia gazeta* (No. 122) dedicated an article to reviewing tendencies in the contemporary literature of Soviet Belarus. An author by the name Pestrak notes that literature is getting very close to the workers there. Young people recently started to 'fancy psychoanalysis', he mentions. He supplied the mention with some gentle, but not too harsh, critique saying about the importance of social reasoning that psychoanalysis lacks. Or in 1967, an article in *Izvestiia* (No. 10) tells a story about the dreams of a university student who is going to become a teacher. He collects in his drawer books by Dostoevsky, Zweig, Kant, and even 'malign' Freud to take with him when he will be assigned to teach in the school.

*Pravda* and *Izvestiia* kept informing Soviet citizens about Freud's life. They announced when Freud's books were burned publicly, when he lost his professorship in Vienna, when he had to escape from the Nazis to London, and news about his death (*Izvestiia*, 1938, No. 67; *Pravda*, 1938, No. 79; *Pravda*,

1938, No. 339; *Izvestiia*, 1939, No. 223). In 1945, the journal *Ogonek* (No. 8) even published an article about the extermination camp Treblinka, a story of how things were done there and the tragic death of Freud's sister Rosa. Frau Freud, on arrival at the camp, proclaims that she is a relative of the famous Prof Sigmund Freud and therefore should be sent to secretarial work or something. The persecutor looks at her documents and reassures her that it was a mistake, and she can even catch the train back to Vienna, but first, she must take a 'bath'. Happily, she undresses and goes to the 'bath'. Later her corpse is found together with everyone else's.

From the mid-1940s the use of Freud's name, or the mention of psychoanalysis without criticism, was much less common. In the 1950s psychoanalysis was linked to American culture and represented imperialism. From the mid-1960s, the word 'psychoanalysis' began to be used as a common noun with a range of meanings:

a   psychoanalysis as a synonym for thinking or self-reflection. That meant if I think or reflect too much about things, I do psychoanalysis;
b   as a synonym for interrogation or assumption. Don't you psychoanalyse me! – one could say;
c   a synonym of understanding hidden motivations and affective states. 'She did psychoanalysis on him', meant that she reflected and understood him;
d   as a synonym of analysis – the process of a detailed examination of something;
e   'performing psychoanalysis' holds the meaning of hesitating as opposed to acting;
f   as a synonym of overthinking or excessive analysis, self-reflection, departed from reality, different from a) by holding a negative connotation;
g   as self-analysis resulting in the understanding of one's mistakes.

This inclusion of 'psychoanalysis' into the vocabulary of the language indicates that psychoanalytic theory did something important for Soviet citizens. My suggestion is that it helped to keep the dimension of reflection and interpretation in mind. Perhaps, it could signify thoughtfulness and critical thinking.

Quite often characters in fictional pieces or translations from foreign literature in *Literaturnaia gazeta* and *Ogonek* mention that they undergo psychoanalysis or read Freud. Frequent references to psychoanalytic treatment started appearing in the late 1960s. In 1960 director Grigori Alexandrov made a comedy Russian Souvenir, where one of the characters, Doctor Adams practices the method of psychoanalysis, that he uses to treat the Italian Duchess (and a spy) for insomnia. Perhaps, the return of Freud and interest in the unconscious of that time in academic circles resulted in the additional public spread of Freud's name.[13]

The knowledge of Freud's texts might be well illustrated by a satirical story, published in *Literaturnaia gazeta* (1970, No. 37). It describes a note from the worker of the factory to the director, explaining why the worker addressed the director by the wrong father's name (otchestvo). Instead of Andrey Viktorovich, he said Andrey Antonovich.

The note presents an analysis – much like the Freudian analysis of the forgotten name of Signorelli, – illustrating how this substitution happened. The analysis is done brilliantly and follows Freud's *The Psychopathology of Everyday Life* (1901) [translation is mine]:

> Dear Andrei Viktorovich!
>
> I want to explain to you the unpleasant incident that occurred between us on the evening of the 7th of this month of this year.
>
> As you remember, this evening, meeting with me at the entrance. You politely nodded to me, to which I also politely said: "Goodbye, Andrei Antonovich", to which you quite rightly remarked; "I, my dear, was always Andrey Viktorovich, not Antonovich..." After which you got into the car and left.
>
> I don't know about you, but for me this unfortunate misunderstanding caused great bitterness and emotional sediment, which has not disappeared so far. It would be strange to think that I did not know or forgot the patronym of my director. It would be even more ridiculous to imagine that by calling you 'Andrei Antonovich', I put some secret meaning into my words or tried to insult you or your father in some way.
>
> It was absolutely not the case, and now, thinking over what happened, I come to the conclusion that my words were the result of a purely subconscious process in the brain, which, using Freud's theory, I will try to explain to you.
>
> An hour before meeting you, I approached our club, where the TV is always on, and found out that Dynamo Moscow was losing to Spartak with a score of 0:2 [football match]. This news upset me very much, a long time Dynamo fan. "Now do not recoup", I thought.
>
> Farewell, victory! The word 'victory' is translated into Latin by the word 'Victoria'. I draw your attention to this stage of my thinking, because from that moment on the word 'Victoria' caused me unpleasant emotions, and according to Freud's theory, my subconscious mind tried to extinguish them to the best of its ability.
>
> In such a state of mind, I approached the checkpoint and suddenly heard the rumble of an airplane above me. The plane is flying, I thought. "Where is it flying, the plane?" My mind was on the plane, I was imagining it flying south, where it's hot right now. But then I remembered the paradoxical fact that in the very, very south of our planet, namely in Antarctica, it is now very cold. "So what if it is cold there?" I thought.
>
> "Isn't it possible to work there too? Don't our whalers under these conditions extract tons of whale oil and whalebone?"

I emphasized these two words: "ANtarctica" and "TONs", because positive, pleasant emotions are connected with these words in my mind, caused by the courageous work of our whalers.

Thus, these two words, the first syllables of which give the name 'ANTON', became fixed in my brain and filled the gap that had formed from the repressed unwanted word 'VICTORIA' (*Literaturnaia gazeta*, 1970, N37, p. 16). How was it possible that in 1970, 40 years after the 'ban' of psychoanalysis and its disappearance, an author of this newspaper knew Freud's work on such a sophisticated level?

## Figurants of the case of the unconscious: Academic discussion of Freud in the Soviet press

This part looks at the press coverage for academic events between 1930 and 1980 to see if there were any other occasions for discussion on Freud or psychoanalysis. Overall findings suggest that the attack on Freudism in the mid-1920s cut short discussion about psychoanalysis for 38 years, but only in academia. There Freud and the unconscious were rehabilitated by the Freud Session in 1958.

*Literaturnaia gazeta* in 1940 (No. 54) published an article by Pyotr Anokhin about new findings in studies on higher nervous activity. There he introduced a new field in physiology, which is serving as a basis for understanding mental disturbances. He said that "what Freud called unconscious is now possible to study scientifically". These views, however, in 10 years costed Anokhin several academic positions, as he was accused of thinking against the only ideologically accepted theory – Pavlovian reflexology. The attack on Freud and the combination of Freudism with reflexology, as well as modern interpretations of Pavlov's theory and public criticism of scientists engaged with foreign ideas, was the main topic of the Pavlov session. This event was of such importance that the script of it was fully published in *Pravda* in 1950 (No. 181 and No. 182). From the full stenograph of the session, we know that Anokhin was one of these scientists who went against Pavlov, distorted his original thinking and mixed with foreign bourgeois theories. We find an echo of this session in *Literaturnaia gazeta* (1952, No. 30) in the critical article, denouncing Dmitry Uznadze for following Freud and rejecting Pavlov, and for his theory of set being idealistic. Three years later, *Pravda* (1953, No. 320) published another portion of the critique of subjectivity in science. Freud is mentioned as a source for physiologists and psychologists who are still not keeping up with Pavlov's theory, so we see that the abandonment of Freud was not immediate.

In the late 1960s and through the 1970s, *Literaturnaia gazeta* published a series of conversations with doctors and psychotherapists, and within them, we find several publications about the unconscious, Freud and psychotherapy.

In *Literaturnaia gazeta* in 1967 (No. 36) a therapist Dr Krelin suggested, that "it is not necessary to accept everything that Freud says, but every doctor should be familiar with psychoanalysis". It is important to note that this was a suggestion he addressed to general practitioners, not psychotherapists or psychiatrists. He continued: "It is necessary to understand the individuality of the patient, however, without psychoanalysis it is difficult to do so". Overall, the article provided a good outline of the psychoanalytic method and indicated the importance of the subjective approach to the patient in general practice, as the mental health of the patient is an important part of physical recovery. Next to this article, we see a polemical response by Snezhnevsky, a psychiatrist, whose name is associated with the abuse of psychiatric power against dissidents. He acknowledged Freud and his popularity in Russia, as well as the value of a psychoanalytic method, but suggested it should be rather studied as a part of the history of psychotherapy, and the method itself cannot offer much to contemporary medicine. The tone of his response, compared to the early year, is soft and Freud was not subjected to many attacks.

Two years later, *Literaturnaia gazeta* (1969, No. 45) published a note by the writer Vladimir Mikhailov titled 'Psychoanalysis: a new religion?' From it, we discover, that by pure chance, Mikhailov arrived in Rome the day after the 26th Psychoanalytic Congress of IPA. (He didn't mention why he was in Rome, and to assume that this was an ordinary trip abroad is rather difficult, because foreign travel was strictly regulated for ordinary Soviet citizens.) The article presents that it happened that Mikhailov 'overheard' a conversation between some young people about psychoanalysis, as he sat in the café next to their table, then he joined their discussion and documented their views. When Mikhailov returned to Moscow he asked Bassin (whose book on the question of the unconscious was published in Moscow a year before) to give a commentary about psychoanalysis. In his response, Bassin affirmed the necessity to return to psychoanalysis and the danger of silencing it.

In subsequent years, the same author Vladimir Mikhailov invited more guests into a conversation about psychotherapy. They discussed neuroses with psychotherapist Boris Karvasarskii[14] (*Literaturnaia gazeta*, 1973, No. 6), and Freud was mentioned as someone who also suggested the connection of neuroses with personality (like Karvasarskii). With Professor Chertok (a French psychotherapist and one of the main speakers in the future 'Symposium on the Unconscious' in Tbilisi in 1978) they discussed psychotherapy and Freud was mentioned as core for psychosomatic medicine (*Literaturnaia gazeta*, 1976, No. 47).

In 1977 *Literaturnaia gazeta* (No. 48) published two materials about the unconscious: an article by A. Prangishvili, the head of the Uznadze Institute in Georgia, and polemics about the Soviet critique of Freud between Harvard Professor Nancy Rollins and Filip Bassin/A. Sherosia. Rollins emphasized the importance of the contribution of Soviet scientists, who argued that unconscious activity is qualitatively different from conscious. Thus, their study of the unconscious is not just a study of non-conscious activity, and this observation is very much in line with my arguments. Overall, a reader can gain a lot of knowledge on the unconscious, repression, sublimation, and psychic defence mechanisms from these pieces. All the Soviet participants of that discussion appeared very soon again in the pages of *Literaturnaia gazeta* (1980, No. 21) in the reportage about the Congress on the Unconscious in Tbilisi. Even though the appearances of Bassin, Uznadze, and Anokhin in the press is a single occurrence, it is nevertheless simultaneously used in the company of Freud's name or the unconscious or psychoanalysis.

The consistent presence of Freud's name in the Soviet press throughout the years 1920–1980, even though framed negatively, provided a vague knowledge of psychoanalysis,[15] which therefore was available for anyone who read newspapers and journals. Freud survived years of attacks and denunciations, and by the beginning of the 1980s, criticism of psychoanalysis became somehow outdated. A new question arose: "Is it necessary to constantly attack Freud?" (*Ogonek*, 1980, No. 37).

## Other clinical directions

As a part of the public dissemination, in this section of the chapter I consider the presence of psychoanalytic ideas in the Soviet clinic, including psychotherapy and general therapy. While we cannot affirm the development of psychoanalytic clinics in the Soviet Union due to the lack of training institutes for future psychoanalysts and absence of private practices, it is still impossible to claim that psychoanalytic knowledge was absent from there.

The split between 'official psychoanalysis' and 'chasing knowledge' opens the space for us to think about the way psychoanalysis existed outside of the binary of training institution knowledge and underground practice – in a form of curiosity that is related to psychoanalytic theory and methodology.[16]

In Soviet Russia training institutes did not have a chance to be established, for multiple reasons. As we have seen already in other chapters, the process of consolidation of science and education in Stalinist times underwent very specific transformations. The establishment of the Psychoanalytic Institute in Moscow was a promising beginning, but short-lived. Altogether, as was previously highlighted by many scholars (Etkind, 1997; Miller, 1998, Rozhdestvenskii, 2009), this was an Institute that was supported by the state, and eventually this engagement served as bad luck for it. Even if psychoanalysis were to be taught, for example, at universities for doctors and psychologists, the whole training system would not work exactly as in the West due to the absence of private practice; one could only meet a psychoanalyst within a state hospital or a day clinic. That, of course, would not prevent doctors or psychologists being curious about psychoanalytic theory and including some elements of it in their psychotherapeutic practice. But this would not exactly be easy either. Psychotherapy as a theory and practice had to undergo the same ideological changes in the Stalinist Era as everything else. The biologization of psychology and the Pavlov campaign, as has already been discussed, provided a different ground for studies of the mind, or, better, to the brain and nervous system. In her study of psychotherapy under Soviet rule, Alexandra Brokman states,

> Psychotherapy that existed in the post-Stalin USSR cannot accurately be described as treatment of the psyche. Although it was understood as acting through it, its influence could be directed at any part of the organism, for example circulatory or digestive system. Consequently, in addition to being an important means of combatting certain disorders affecting the mind, psychotherapy was seen as applicable in treatment of a variety of somatic symptoms, and its practitioners stressed its potential to improve the functioning of the entire organism.
> 
> (Brokman, 2018, p. 22)

For a moment this might look like a perfect combination: psyche was considered in its unity with the body, and that could actually enrich psychotherapeutic practice. However, Brokman observes that on the top of the whole organism Soviet psychotherapy put the will "which was portrayed as capable of governing and reshaping both the body and the patterns of thinking, emotions, and personality traits that composed the mind" (2018, p. 23). Related to this, the idea of self-improvement rather than self-understanding is crucial in her work, summarizing that psychotherapy in the Soviet Union could not be separated from the ideological push towards becoming a hero. As Brokman notices, psychotherapists did not address the wider public. Instead, their efforts to promote treatment were focused on healthcare authorities and administrators in charge. In other words, the struggle of psychotherapy in the Soviet Union was mostly ideological. Certainly, treatment in such circumstances was about finding the power of words to persuade the patient's mind the right way. This shift from internal to external in psychotherapy represents the dynamic of the communist state, where one did not count without being part of the bigger whole. Thus, inevitably, we can observe the split between theory and practice. No matter how wholesome or advanced the theory of the mind was, if free association technique was eventually to lose out to suggestive techniques, psychoanalysis as a practice would not survive. And so psychotherapy could not develop not because of the insufficiency of theory, but because of ideological constraints.

Similar changes in psychiatry had started already in 1936 after the decree on pedological perversions. In his study on psychiatry in Stalinist times, Benjamin Zajicek traces various shifts that ideology produced. "Biomedical scientists, in short, were warned away from claiming special expertise in detecting and treating social problems" (Zajicek, 2009, p. 3). Even though psychiatry was not mentioned directly, since that year psychiatry should have been only focused on the medical treatment of ill patients (p. 5). Illnesses included major psychoses and diseases of the central nervous system (p. 6). The notion of 'social', thus, was excluded from psychiatric discourse.

If in 1930 there was still a discussion of mental hygiene and the role of psychiatry in building the new society, helping to promote mental health and social support for citizens (Zajicek, 2009, p. 3–4), during the Second Five Year Plan (1933–1937) all sorts of fatigue and reactions of people to social and physical hardship was outside of psychiatric interest.

> Under Stalinism, psychiatrists were to have professional jurisdiction over people suffering from specific disease entities, conditions that were qualitatively different from normal health. Fatigue, headaches, problems of social adjustment, and other 'normal' reactions to difficulty were to be the jurisdiction of industrial managers, teachers, and Party activists, not psychiatric professionals. The job of psychiatrists was to study and treat specific mental diseases, not to study and treat the society as whole.
> (Zajicek, 2014, p. 181)

Shock therapy, electroshock, and lobotomy as biological methods were introduced in the aftermath of 1936. Unlike in psychotherapy, however, this ideological intervention transformed not a practice only, but also a theory. Gradually, the classification of mental 'illnesses' relied more and more on theories of biological genetic imbalance or derivatives of nervous system typologies. Of course, interest in psychoanalysis did not vanish completely from the clinical scene because of that, and there is occasional evidence of psychiatrists, psychotherapists and psychologists practicing it.[17] However, due to the impossibility of psychoanalysis to receive official status in Soviet Union, due to major shifts in psychotherapy and psychiatry in the 1930s, as well as absence of training institutes, the only way that the dissemination of psychoanalysis could take place is as a form of knowledge. This knowledge belonged both to the public and to academic circles. As my next chapters will show, this knowledge continued to infiltrate the work of psychologists of the old generation, like Zeigarnik, Uznadze and Luria. An active disseminator of this knowledge after 1958, Bassin attempted and partially succeeded in bringing it to a younger generation of psychologists too.

## Notes

1 Witness history. No sex in the USSR. www.bbc.co.uk/sounds/play/p0574s3p
2 It is important to note that before then women technically were property, e.g., did not have individual rights. For a detailed account on social changes and women liberation see Goldman (1993).
3 Quote from Omel'chenko (2000) p. 141.
4 In contrast, 'gestalt' has only two matches in the whole period 1900-1980, 'behaviourism' – 13. To conduct the research for 'hypnosis' and 'unconscious' was impossible because these words are used outside of the clinical language, so to distinguish between relevant and irrelevant use in the context of the present research was impossible.

5 *Pravda* [Truth] was the official voice of Soviet communism and the Central Committee of the Communist Party between 1918 and 1991. Founded in 1912 in St. Petersburg, *Pravda* originated as an underground daily workers' newspaper and was subjected to constant persecution, fines, penalties, and prohibitions by the government. To avoid censorship and forced closures, the name of the newspaper changed multiple times during its early years. Before long, however, *Pravda* became the main newspaper of the revolutionary wing of the Russian socialist movement. Throughout the Soviet era, party members were obligated to read *Pravda*. Today, *Pravda* remains the official organ of the Communist Party of the Russian Federation, an important political faction in contemporary Russian politics (EastView description).

6 Among the longest-running Russian newspapers, *Izvestiia* [News] was founded in March 1917 and during the Soviet period was the official organ of the Presidium of the Supreme Soviet of the USSR. Remarkable for its serious and balanced treatment of subject matter, *Izvestiia* has traditionally been a popular news source within intellectual and academic circles. Continuously published for over 100 years, *Izvestiia's* prominence endures today as one of the most subscribed news sources of contemporary Russia, covering domestic and foreign policy, commentary, culture, education, and finance (EastView description).

7 Established on April 22, 1929 with the support of the "father of Soviet literature", writer Maxim Gorky, *Literaturnaia gazeta* [Literary Newspaper] is a landmark publication in Russia's cultural heritage. With its focus on literary and intellectual life, *Literaturnaia gazeta* allowed Soviet Russia's preeminent authors, poets, and cultural figures a podium for commentary, affording perhaps fewer restrictions than might be possible in other publications. In 1932 *Literaturnaia gazeta* became the official organ of the Union of Soviet Writers, the government-run organization which controlled most literary publications and the employment of writers in the USSR. In the post-World War II period, the scope of *Literaturnaia gazeta* expanded from an exclusively literary newspaper to more of a literary, social and political publication, becoming one of the most authoritative and influential publications in the country. As one of the most open newspapers of the Soviet era, *Literaturnaia gazeta* was truly significant in the cultural life of the Soviet Union, and remains popular among the intelligentsia in today's Russia (EastView description).

8 *Kul'tura* [Culture], as it is known today, is the most important Soviet and Russian publication on culture from 1929 to the present, with reviews of major events in literature, theatre, cinematography and arts. For nearly 100 years, *Kul'tura* has provided a unique perspective on ever-changing attitudes toward arts and culture in Soviet and Russian societies. *Kul'tura* was previously published as *Rabochii i iskusstvo* (Workers and Art, 1929–1930), *Sovetskoe iskusstvo* (Soviet Art, 1931–1941), *Literatura i iskusstvo* (Literature and Art, 1942–1944), *Sovetskoe iskusstvo* (1944–1953), and *Sovetskaia kul'tura* (Soviet Culture, 1953–1991).

*Rabochii i iskusstvo* was established during a time when artists had relative freedom to create works for the New Soviet man. Artists were enthusiastic in spreading the socialist revolution, and the newspaper at this time reflects that mindset. During the Stalin years, Socialist realism took hold. Any creative expression considered unworthy to support the goals of socialism and communism was banned. Writers such as Mikhail Zoshchenko, Osip Mandelstam, Boris Pasternak, and others were roundly criticized in the pages of *Sovetskoe iskusstvo, Literatura i iskusstvo*, and *Sovetskoe iskusstvo*.

*Sovetskaia kul'tura*, established in 1953, came about in the thaw of the Khrushchev era. The times changed for the better, but the newspaper still toed the party line. Modern art exhibitions were condemned and avant-garde composers and abstract painters were censured. During the Gorbachev era, *glasnost* created a cultural reawakening, which was reflected in the pages of *Sovetskaia kul'tura*. For example, the newspaper was the first to report that authorities had rehabilitated Pasternak posthumously and a museum dedicated to the work of Marc Chagall was to open in Belarus. Today, the newspaper offers interesting reviews and event listings, often focusing on the cultural life of Moscow and the regions. It is also known for its topical commentaries on popular culture and politics (EastView description).

9 The history of the satirical magazine *Krokodil* [Crocodile] goes back to 1922, when it first appeared as a supplement to *Rabochaia Gazeta* (formerly *Rabochii*) under the direction of its editor Yeremeev. K.S. The growing popularity and circulation of *Rabochaia Gazeta*, combined with the fact that many satirical voices were present in the widening pool of talented journalists, led the editors of the newspaper to establish on June 4, 1922 a separate satirical issue to be circulated free of charge to the subscribers of the newspaper.

The newly established supplementary issue satirized a host of issues and holdovers from pre- revolutionary Russia, including White Russian emigres, the Orthodox Church, bourgeois intellectuals, as well as diverse groups of social outcasts (moonshiners, black marketeers, etc.). After a three-month period of largely haphazard satirical writing, the supplement found its stride and honed its method of bringing its readers incisive satirical commentary. The success of the experiment among its growing readership would directly lead to the establishment of *Krokodil* as a separate publication on August 27, 1922.

Published continuously until 2008, *Krokodil* was at one time the most popular magazine for humorous stories and satire, with a circulation reaching 6.5 million copies. *Krokodil* lampooned religion, alcoholism, foreign political figures and events. It ridiculed bureaucracy and excessive centralized control. The caricatures found in *Krokodil* can be studied as a gauge of the 'correct party line' of the time. During the height of the Cold War, cartoons criticizing Uncle Sam, Pentagon, Western colonialism and German militarism were common in the pages of *Krokodil* (EastView description).

10 *Ogonek* [Spark, or twinkle] was one of the oldest weekly magazines in Russia, having been in continuous publication since 1923. Throughout its illustrious history *Ogonek* published original works by such Soviet cultural luminaries as Vladimir Mayakovsky, Isaac Babel, Ilya Ilf and Evgeny Petrov, Yevgeny Yevtushenko, the photographer Yuri Rost, and others. It first saw the rise of its stock under the editorial guidance of Mikhail Koltsov, a star Soviet reporter, who oversaw the growth of *Ogonek* from a readership of 25,000 in 1923 to nearly half a million within a mere two-year period, turning it into one of the most influential and widely read Soviet publications of the period. Its popularity was left intact even after Koltsov's arrest on the eve of the WWII in 1938. It is safe to say however, that the magazine would not have become the cultural force it was but for the editorial tenure of Anatoli Sofronov, the noted Soviet poet and playwright. Under Sofronov's at times controversial and at times bromidic leadership, Ogonek became an important outlet for some of the most well-known and respected Soviet writers, visual artists, photographers and reporters. Although under Sofronov *Ogonek* grew steadily, it came to experience the peak of its popularity at the hands of its new editor Vitaly Korotich, who assumed editorship of the magazine after the passing of Sofronov in 1986 at the height of Perestroika. Korotich, inspired by the newfound political liberties, turned the journal into a lively space for edgy political commentary, criticism, and satire (EastView description).

11 The clinical presence of psychoanalysis will be discussed in more detail in the third part of this chapter.

12 This argument will be strengthened in the chapter about Luria, by the discussion of some archival documents, related to Luria's doctorate dissertation defence and award of the degree of doctor of psychology.

13 Also circulated in the form of anecdotes, for example, from *Krokodil*:
"A fashionable psychiatrist sits in a bar and with a grim look drinks whisky.
Listen – the drinking companion tells him. – You are even more depressed than your patients. Why don't you psychoanalyse yourself?
I can't! – He answers with a sob in his voice. – My services are too expensive" (1966, No. 25).

14 A pupil of Miasishchev and for many years the Head of the Bekhterev Psycho-neurological Institute in Leningrad and then in Saint-Petersburg. Karvasarskii is known for his 'own' method of psychotherapy, which originated in Miasishchev's idea of the importance of the 'system of relations' of the individual for mental health and therapy.

15 The specific interest in psychoanalysis among non-psychologists or psychiatrists was also present throughout these years. A brief search through an archive of diaries of the Soviet people, collected in the project 'Prozhito' https://prozhito.org, shows that to some extent knowledge of Freud, attempts at self-analysis, academic discussions and conversations with friends about psychoanalysis all got some space in the diary entries.

16 Pointing to the impact in the West of the regulations growing within psycho-analysis in the first quarter of the 20th century, Forrester noted, "but as the definition of 'official' psychoanalysis came into focus in the mid-1920s, with the rules governing training, qualification and the overall aim of psychoanalytic institutions, such larger-than-life natives of the 'scientific' world would find it less easy to include psychoanalysis in their public preoccupations – although many of them would, naturally, continue to end up on the couch. Did the rise of 'official' psychoanalysis put an end to such promiscuous pursuing of knowledge?" (Cameron and Forrester, 2017, p. 430).

17 Zajicek notes that among other forms of psychotherapy, psychoanalysis was practiced by some doctors during the war in 1942 (2009, p. 148). Olga Arnold, a former pupil of Filipp Bassin, remembers that in 1970s "At the Department of Psychotherapy at the Institute for Advanced Training of Doctors (TsOLIUV), in the Psychiatric Hospital number 12th and in the crisis centre, all psychotherapists were familiar with psychoanalytic theory, we used certain methods of psychoanalysis in our work" (From email exchange, November 2021). She also remembers that Prof Vladimir Rozhnov in the early 1970s was reading lectures on psychoanalysis. This corresponds to the information provided in the encyclopaedia *Russian Psycho-analysts* (2000) by V. Ovcharenko. There he also brings around 200 names of people who were involved, either in practice or theory, or institutional support of psychoanalysis in Russia, predominantly in the Soviet period. For example, Boris Kravtsov, who started practicing psychoanalysis in the 1960s and created a study group in the 1970s, organized the Doctor's Psychotherapeutic Association (pp. 91–92). His students Sergei Agrachev and Igor Kadyrov were organizers of the Moscow Psychoanalytic Society, which is now a member of IPA and EPF.

Chapter 3

# Zeigarnik, Luria and Vygotsky
Building pathopsychology

This chapter offers a closer look at work of Bluma Zeigarnik and her collaboration with Lev Vygotsky and Alexander Luria.

The theory of pathopsychology and the diagnostic procedure of the 'pathopsychological experiment' that Zeigarnik developed in the Soviet period of her career is in the focus of my analysis and revision. While it is not 'psychoanalysis', it clearly continues the psychoanalytic tradition of research into the psyche. It shares the theoretical understanding of mental processes, as well as the origin of symptoms, which is coherent with Luria and Vygotsky's take on psychoanalysis. Also, their approach to schizophrenia is seen in this chapter as an alternative to the official psychiatry of that time, which abused the diagnosis 'schizophrenia' for the purposes of the control and persecution of dissent. The way schizophrenia was seen and treated by Zeigarnik and her pupils is closer to contemporary psychoanalytic understanding of it.

It is important to note, however, that Zeigarnik never openly claimed to be a psychoanalyst or advocated for practicing psychoanalysis, and in her way was sceptical of psychotherapy in general, focusing instead on the potential of pathopsychology to become a tool for successful rehabilitation in the hands of clinical psychologists. This could be due to political reasons, this could be genuine repudiation of psychoanalysis, and I am not going to speculate which was the truth. Thus, in this chapter I do not claim that psychoanalytic ideas were dominant in Zeigarnik's work or see her as a follower of psychoanalysis. Nonetheless, I suggest that the encounter with psychoanalysis for Zeigarnik was not without consequences, and that her mention of Freud in her writings was not just a result of her erudition but also served wider conceptual purposes. Indeed, her continuous mentioning of Freud in her writings, both in the form of reference and critique, helped keep psychoanalytic theory alive as a subject of discussion through the years of its prohibition. In the light of recent examinations of the parallels between the ideas of Vygotsky and Lacan (Zavershneva, 2019), Vygotsky and Winnicott (Orozco, 2021) and Luria and Freud (Solms, 2000), Zeigarnik's theoretical ability to adopt and adapt psychoanalytic understanding of mental disturbances, as well as to maintain a 'psychoanalytic position' towards the patient within the institutional setting, makes her a good candidate to be included in the history of psychoanalysis in Soviet Russia as one of the vicissitudes.

Following the general line of current study, which is a historical and theoretical exploration, this chapter navigates between historical testimonies and subjective interpretation and seeks to explore ways of reading Zeigarnik's heritage. Since the archival evidence is poor, her texts become especially important as representatives of her theoretical views in the Soviet period of her career. While I am aware of the interpretative nature of my suggestions, it is nevertheless done in line with a series of social-historical studies of life in Soviet Russia, and with work on Soviet psychology and the history of psychoanalysis. In common with some contemporary psychosocial research methods, I also employ psychoanalytic attentiveness to details and inconsistencies when reading Zeigarnik's texts.

## The unfinished history of Zeigarnik

Zeigarnik is not referenced in English-language studies of the history of Soviet psychology and Soviet science (Kozulin, 1984; Joravsky, 1989; Graham, 1988), nor on the history of psychoanalysis (Etkind, 1997; Miller, 1998), though there is a brief mention of Zeigarnik's work included in the revisionist study of Vygotsky (Yasnitsky and van der Veer, 2015). In English, there are several articles dedicated to her life and work that emphasize her role in the establishment of Russian clinical psychology (Nikolaeva, 2011; Marko, 2018; MacLeod, 2020). Zeigarnik's name is well-known, however, by a wide range of clinicians in the mental health field in Russia and other post-Soviet countries. The pathopsychological experiment that she invented regularly forms the basis for work by clinical psychologists in psychiatric hospitals or day clinics. Her findings are widely used for diagnosis and differential diagnosis, and her book *Pathopsychology* (1969 and multiple editions) is the classic handbook for clinical psychology students. None of these sources explore the possible engagement with psychoanalytic theory by Zeigarnik or the methodological continuity of Soviet psychology with psychoanalysis among Vygotsky and Luria's disciples.

References to Zeigarnik's name can be found in many psychoanalytic articles and books (Szasz, 1958; Silbermann, 1961; Spitz, 1964; Lagache, 1950, 1951; Schur, 1966; Lacan, 1991; Etchegoyen, 1999; Nobus, 2000; Hill, 2002; Fink, 2017; Hook, 2017) in relation to her experimental discovery from her pre-Soviet career, called the Zeigarnik effect.[1] Although in these texts she has been, on occasion, cited as a man or given the wrong first name, her contribution to the understanding of transference and dreamwork and the work of memory, fetishism, the construction of the ego, and traumatic repetition is highly valued. Despite this, her later work from the Soviet period of her career (1930–80s), for example, her research on thought disturbances and schizophrenia, is not discussed at all.

One possible explanation for Zeigarnik's omission from historical studies may be the lack of archival material that references her. What we know about her life is sourced mostly from the memoirs of her grandson Andrei (A. Zeigarnik, 2001), and memoirs of her disciples (Nikolaeva, 2003; Zolotova, 2007, 2016; Nikovaeva and Poliakov, 2016). Some details of her professional life can be found in studies on Vygotsky (Yasnitsky and van der Veer, 2015; Zavershneva and van der Veer, 2017). Even the family archive is poor, as most of her personal papers were confiscated when her husband was accused of espionage for Germany. With great danger to herself and her two sons, Zeigarnik spent many years trying to appeal against his sentence without success. Former disciples and colleagues recall that this shocking experience made her a very private person, who rarely shared details of her life and beliefs ('Zeiigarnikovskie chteniia', 2020). So, her consequent development of an 'internal censorship' further affected her archive (A. Zeigarnik, 2001).

However, there might be another explanation for Zeigarnik's omission: the historiographical tradition of Soviet and Russian psychology, which Yasnitsky (2015) suggests formulating as a reproduction of the 'Stalinist model'. In his view, this historiographical tradition claims the presence of unique and original features within Soviet psychology. Such a claim to originality requires what Yasnitsky calls a 'hagiographic tradition in historiography', aiming at reproductions of narratives supporting the unique status of Soviet psychological theories, affirming their isolationism.[2] Applied to the history of Zeigarnik, this tradition necessarily isolates her from foreign theories. In cases where the possibility of influence is undeniable, such as that of Gestalt theory – because Zeigarnik worked in Berlin with Kurt Lewin – other possible theoretical influences are excluded in order to maintain the status of Zeigarnik as an 'original' Soviet psychologist.

The growing field of the studies of 'psy-disciplines' in the Soviet bloc (Zajicek, 2009; Savelli and Marks, 2015; Reich, 2018; Brokman, 2018) shows how various theoretical schools continued to be present under communist regimes and describes the challenges that Soviet psychologists had to endure to continue their practices. While prominent figures of Soviet psychology such as Vygotsky and Luria have had their work reviewed and rethought, including in regard to their relationships with psychoanalysis after 1930 (Proctor, 2020; Cole, 2006; Solms, 2000; Yasnitsky, 2015; van der Veer and Zavershneva, 2017; Hames, 2002), Bluma Zeigarnik was one of many women psychologists whose name is somehow omitted from revisionist research on Soviet psychology, despite having worked closely with Luria and Vygotsky. At least two more names, Gita Birenbaum and Susanna Rubinstein should be added to the list of the prominent Soviet women psychologists. The role of women in Soviet science is yet to be researched in more detail.

## Bluma Zeigarnik and Soviet psychology, 1930–80s[3]

In this section of the chapter I return to the 'roots' of Luria and Vygotsky's ideas in order to provide the context for Zeigarnik's arrival in Moscow. While she worked in Berlin under the supervision of Kurt Lewin and was undoubtedly influenced by his ideas and the way he conducted his experiments, teachers who Zeigarnik met in Moscow and who had a great interest in psychoanalysis have not previously been included in the picture of her theoretical background.

### Luria, Vygotsky and psychoanalysis

As a young enthusiast of psychoanalysis and future teacher and colleague of Bluma Zeigarnik, Alexander Luria founded the Kazan Psychoanalytic Group (1921) and became secretary of the All-Russian Psychoanalytic Society when he moved to Moscow (1923). His future colleague Lev Vygotsky – the second Soviet teacher of Zeigarnik – was also involved in meetings of the Psychoanalytic Society, although he was not a member. As Etkind claims in his study, psychoanalyst Sabina Spielrein might have had an influence on both Luria and Vygotsky, especially her paper 'Aphasic and Infantile Thought'.[4] That is to suggest that aphasia, child development, the role of language for thinking – leading scientific interests for both Luria and Vygotsky – could have been formed in their acquaintance with psychoanalysis. In addition to Spielrein being a possible and unacknowledged influence on Vygotsky's and Piaget's works (Santiago-Delefosse and Delefosse, 2002), there are multiple similarities and references that support the view that Vygotsky and Piaget were influenced by psychoanalysis (Cordón, 2012). These include the similarity and methodological agreement between Freud's (1891) and Luria's (1947) classification of aphasia (Solms, 2000); multiple references to Freud's ideas in their early work; most importantly, Luria's 'Psychoanalysis as a System of Monistic Psychology' (1925) and Luria's and Vygotsky's 'Preface to the Russian Translation of *Beyond the Pleasure Principle*' (1925), and the claim that it was actually Vygotsky who translated it (Santiago-Delefosse and Delefosse, 2002).[5]

However, as discussed in previous chapters, political changes including the rise of Stalin created circumstances for the ideological suppression of psychoanalysis.[6] Considering the political campaign against psychoanalysis, we should question the nature of Luria and Vygotsky's criticism of psychoanalysis, especially when it appears in the 1930s.

As for Zeigarnik, it is uncertain if her critique was a way to keep Freud in her texts or a genuinely critical position. The debate around what Soviet people believed and practised has several positions, and I rely here on a view outside of the binary opposition between a 'true believer' and a 'dissident', which is presented in work done around humour in Stalin's times (Waterlow, 2018), and everyday life in late socialism (Yurchak, 2005). Such activity was not a consciously anti-state position. I see the engagement with Freud through the lens of historical continuities in the career of Russian psychologists including Zeigarnik. Luria's and Bassin's active interest in psychoanalysis in the 1920s did not change dramatically after the 1930s, even though they had to change their theoretical vocabulary and engage with medicine and physiology. Therefore, in their later work, we can still find links to their earlier ideas, enriched by interdisciplinary research. My view is that Zeigarnik enjoyed a similar continuity and that her interests continued to be explored throughout the years, despite the censorship and interruptions of dangerous times. This conveys a possibility of identity, distinct from the dichotomy of 'totalitarian self' or being dissident, as drawn for example by Anna Krylova (2000) in her critique of such narratives about Soviet identities.

It is worth emphasising that Zeigarnik moved to Soviet Moscow when she was 30, as a mature scientist with already existing international fame. In the same vein, her closest colleagues Luria and Vygotsky formed their scientific interests in the international spirit and freedom of the first decade after the October Revolution. The transformations of the 1930s and hardships of the 1940s were rather traumatic for her and resulted in self-censorship. For a new generation, born in the 1930s, perhaps, to engage with Freud, who was against the law, might have been a kind of protest activity in the late 1960s, while to the older generation it was a question of self- continuity as researchers. Thus, I treat it not as an issue of identity, but as an issue of finding ways for researchers such as Zeigarnik to practice according to their longstanding interests. Let's look closer at Zeigarnik's life and career.

### Zeigarnik's early years

Full biographical details of Bluma Zeigarnik are available for the English reader in the memoirs of her grandson Andrei Zeigarnik (2001) and presented also in Marko (2018) and MacLeod (2020). I will focus only on some episodes of her professional biography to contextualize her theoretical and clinical development. Zeigarnik was born in Lithuania in a Jewish family. She moved to Berlin to study and only later in life moved to Soviet Moscow, following her husband, who got a post there.

Zeigarnik's career as a psychologist began in 1924. She attended seminars led by Kurt Lewin at Berlin University and soon joined his team to conduct experiments in his laboratory. She received her doctoral degree in 1927 and published the results of an experiment on the effect of unfinished tasks on memory – the 'Zeigarnik effect', which was only translated and published in Russian in 2001, as part of Kurt Lewin's works.[7] In 1931 she moved to Moscow and become a colleague of Vygotsky and worked at the Institute of Higher Nervous Activity. In 1935 she was awarded the Candidate of Biological Sciences academic degree, as it was becoming increasingly unsafe to work under degrees from outside Soviet Russia.

## Vygotsky's influence

From Zeigarnik's grandson's memoirs, it is clear that she admired Vygotsky and his work (A. Zeigarnik, 2001). In *Vygotsky's Notebooks*, and in personal letters to colleagues and friends, there are a significant number of references to their collaboration (Zavershneva and van der Veer, 2018).

When Zeigarnik arrived in Moscow, Vygotsky was working on questions of language and its relationship to thinking. Luria's expeditions to Uzbekistan (1931 and 1932)[8] where he studied the development of thinking, complemented and supplemented Vygotsky's theory and led to several interesting conclusions. For example, Luria discovered that Uzbekistani people have no concept of the circle, "instead of the word 'circle' they use words such as 'moon', 'money', 'bowl', 'wheel' and all these forms designate the fact that it is not the perception of the form, but the perception of the meaning" that matters (Zavershneva and van der Veer, 2018, p. 178). At the same time, spots in the Rorschach test, a normal example of the gestalt ability to perceive a circle, were perceived as meaningless for them (p. 178). It became central for Vygotsky's idea that thoughts exist only in the structure of language. For this: (1) perception, (2) language, and (3) thinking were the main components of his theory and objects of his study. These ideas were at the core of Zeigarnik's research. At that time she was exploring changes in thinking and language in psychosis under Vygotsky's supervision (p. 319). His 'semic method'[9] (p. 291) formed the core conceptual components of Zeigarnik's pathopsychology; his notion of a 'zone of proximal development' was a target for clinical evaluation in many of the diagnostic procedures of pathopsychology (Nikolaeva, 2011). His statement about the connection of affect to thinking also found its direct parallel in the classification of thought disturbances developed by Zeigarnik and colleagues.

As Zavershneva and van der Veer (2018) points out, the 'semic method' was never conceptualized in Vygotsky's theoretical writings, but from his notebooks reading they suggest that "the semic method meant the study of *the inner structure of sign operations*, i.e., the analysis of mental phenomena based on their meaning rather than on their external characteristics" (p. 291). The inner structure of sign operations, as follows from the content of Vygotsky's notes organizes the whole consciousness and can explain the nature of it. It is not just verbal acts, or intellectual acts of behaviour that involves speech (p. 291) that interests Vygotsky. His attempt is to understand how words that we acquire structure us as humans. That includes the meaning we make of the world and the self, motivations for actions and emotional states.

In 1932, Vygotsky writes "Meaning is the highest problem of the sign operations. Just like there is no higher behaviour without the sign (without the function of the sign), there is no psychological system without meaning"

(Zavershneva and van der Veer, 2018, p. 301). The problem Vygotsky is trying to solve comes from his findings that the meaning here is not assigned by the meaning of the word only and can vary depending on the personal meaning that is attached to the word. The variation can be of an associative kind but can be just 'random' and linked to the sound image of the word, rather than its written version, it can change depending on the concrete circumstances the person is in, and it can be played around in jokes and poetry. Two examples of shifts of meanings he brings in his notes stood out for me.

The first, a note about the dependency of understanding upon the situation:

> I specify a telegram. By telephone [I dictate] the sender: Vygotsky. 'With Victor?' – I hear: he kicked her, still stricter, constrictor?
> 
> (p. 299)

The second,

> 1. I can forget *what* I wanted to say or about what I wanted to speak: (a) or simply not say what I wanted to say, i.e., forget my intention; (b) remember that I wanted to say *something* but forget *what*.
> 2. Forget the *word*, how it is called what I want to say (corrosion of metal).
> 3. Forget how I wanted to develop this theme – *using which meanings.*
> 
> (p. 300, Vygotsky's emphases)

We can see what could interest Vygotsky in psychoanalysis. For those familiar with Freud's metapsychology, especially the work *The Unconscious* (1915) and importantly its Appendix, the meaning of the inner structure of sign operations. There, Freud suggests that the acquisition of words at first relates to their sound image, and we have no signs until the written form of the word has been learnt, but we have a link between the sound image and the object. He distinguishes between word presentation and thing presentation. In fact, in the notebook from 1926, which Vygotsky filled with ideas on the origin and the function of the speech, he references Freud's idea on the link between the word and the consciousness, and that we cannot know about the unconscious unless words are attached to the unconscious presentations (Zavershneva and van der Veer, 2018, pp. 106–107, 113).

Part of the research Vygotsky did to explore the inner structure of sign operations in 1932 in *Vsesouznyi Institut Eksperimental'noi Mediciny* [All-Soviet Institute of Experimental Medicine] was a study of schizophrenia. Vygotsky's hypothesis was that the core of disturbance in schizophrenia is the "disintegration of meaning of words" (Zeigarnik, 1962, p. 466). Also in *Vygotsky's Notebooks* (Zevershneva, van der Veer, 2017) we find a note that in Luria's family archive there are documents from 1932–1933 with plans for 'experimental' studies based on the 'semic method' (p. 342), partially realized by Zeigarnik and Luria in what will be further discussed as methods of pathopsychology, the method of classification and understanding of proverbs. The disintegration of meaning here, as we now understand, is not related to the cognitive inability, but rather to the domination of the subjective meaning or random meaning or meaning dominated by the sound image of the word over the conventional meaning. This idea will be at the core of the thought disturbance classification proposed by Zeigarnik.

Many years later, in conversation with the Soviet historian of psychology Mikhail Yaroshevsky, Zeigarnik admitted Lewin's influence on her structure of the pathopsychological experiment, but, as a theoretical basis for pathopsychology, Zeigarnik drew on Vygotsky's ideas (Yaroshevsky, 1988). Overall, we find references to Freud in *Vygotsky's Notebooks* in abundance, and it would be difficult to imagine that Freudian ideas escaped Zeigarnik's sight when working with Vygotsky.

### Life without Vygotsky: Luria's co-operation

Prior to Zeigarnik's arrival in Moscow, Luria was conducting a series of experiments (1923–1930) with criminals, university students undergoing examinations, children etc.[10] Results were published under the title *The Nature of Human Conflicts* in 1932 in English and only in 2002 in Russian. In the preface to the Russian publication, Michael Cole explains such a gap with several reasons, among which are Luria's references to Freud and Jung. He also emphasizes that acknowledgement of Luria's interest in psychoanalysis is important in order to be able to understand the book. He notes that, although it was only in his early career that Luria engaged with psychoanalysis openly, "his interest was bigger than just a passing infatuation" (Cole in Luria, 2002, p. 9).

Luria's experiments were structured around finding a method to study mental disturbances as continuing the tradition of the study of mind established by Freud and Jung. His dissatisfaction with the associative method invented by Jung brought him to the new combined motor method (Luria, 2002, p. 37). It is likely that Zeigarnik was familiar with these experiments and discussed them with Luria. She shared with him an interest in finding an experimental basis for the theory of mental disturbances. Luria's method of the evaluation of thinking was included in the standard protocol for the pathopsychological experiment and it is apparent that his other work shaped Zeigarnik's theoretical views, because he is often referenced in her writing. It is easy to imagine that Luria's interest in developing psychoanalysis could have played a part in Zeigarnik's work too.

Luria's work *The Nature of the Human Conflicts* is discussed in more detail in the chapter entitled 'The Criminal' in Proctor's book (2020). There she shows how psychoanalytic theory was embedded in criminology and associative techniques involved in the development of a predecessor of the polygraph machine. The devastation caused by the Revolution had resulted in a wave of crime, and the details of criminal acts available to Luria often seemed senseless:

> a baker accused of killing his wife; a man found in a pile of snow having been hit with a sledgehammer; a factory worker who broke a window at his workplace to steal a ventilator; a man who killed his fiancée and threw her dead body into water tied to a cast-iron wheel" etc.
>
> (p. 48).

Luria's ambition was to incorporate psychoanalytic theory into his work as a Soviet psychologist, even though it was to criminals rather than patients that he turned. Proctor notices, though, that Luria's focus was on whether rather than on why the people he observed had committed murder, pointing, perhaps, to the limits of his analytic capacity. In her view, Luria consequently failed to reflect on the role of the social order in fostering criminal behaviour, being focused instead only on the application of psychological theories, and in experimental proofs of his associative technique. To Proctor, Luria's departure from psychoanalysis was primarily a consequence of the fact that his psychological approach was never primarily psychoanalytic. In Luria's defence, this lack of social reflection may have derived from his own need to shield himself from the devastating loss and disruption which accompanied the post-Revolutionary years. Alongside came general tendencies of erasure of 'social' reasoning in psy-disciplines. Besides, between the 1920s, a period of active involvement in the psychoanalytic movement in Russia and the publication of *The Nature of Human Conflicts* in 1932, significant changes occurred. Growing attacks on psychoanalysis continued as attacks on Luria. In the late 1930s, a period when calling Freud by his name was equated with high treason, Luria lost both of his foundations – psychology and psychoanalysis, and also lost his dear colleague Vygotsky. He found shelter in medicine and specialized in a new object – the brain – which was, however, never primarily a biological substance to him. Luria's work on the brain kept its distance from dry neurological language and instead, as Proctor notes, "Luria composed the text in a self-consciously literary style"[11] (Proctor, 2020, p. 166).

When, in 1940, Zeigarnik's husband was arrested and charged with spying for Germany, it was a dangerous time for her, as anyone could be sentenced for treason or for being a foreign agent. For similar reasons between 1940–1943 Zeigarnik and Luria worked in the town of Kisegach, in their voluntary exile from Moscow.[12] There they researched the causes and consequences of brain damage and experimented on how to restore the lost functions of soldiers with head wounds. During the period of biologization in the country, Luria and Zeigarnik found refuge in studying the psychological effects of brain damage. The full details of their work were never published for ideological reasons (A. Zeigarnik, 2001) as well as for the fact that their research was far from biological. As Zeigarnik formulated it later:

> The theory of the existence of inborn, isolated functions ... assume that for each specific mental function there exists a separate brain centre, and that a lesion of this area causes the disturbance of that function.... We merely note that ... these investigators arrive at oversimplified psycho-morphological correlations.
> (Zeigarnik, 1965, p. 21).

After their return to Moscow, Zeigarnik and Luria remained life-long colleagues and friends. Moreover, their theoretical work remains dedicated to general psychological questions such as thinking and memory, as well as more specific clinical categories like aphasia, schizophrenia, and their overall relation to the regulating role of language.

Luria's trip to London in 1957, where he spent two weeks invited by London University and The British Psychological Society to give lectures, is apparent evidence that the regulating role of language was one of the constant interests in his work. From Luria's report[13] we know that he gave there three lectures at London University titled 'On the role of speech in organisation of normal and abnormal behaviour' and two speeches at The British Psychological Society, titled 'Scientific approach to main forms of abnormal development of the child' and 'Objective analysis of the dynamic of semantic connotations'. Luria also visited the Maudsley Hospital and shared the current research done by Soviet pathopsychologists with clinical psychologists there. In Cambridge he gave a paper on the role of language in regulation of mental functions. In this research we can see echo of Vygotsky's 'semic method' and search for the inner structure of sign operations and regulatory function of the words.

In 1969, Zeigarnik and Luria attended the XIX International Congress of Psychology in London. There Zeigarnik chaired a section on abnormal psychology, and Luria gave a lecture titled 'The Origin and Cerebral Organization of Man's Conscious Action'. In this paper he again demonstrated that his views were more complex and beyond a study of the physiological specifics of the brain. For Luria, "the child's conscious action is originally *divided between two persons*"[14] (p. 4). When mother says "that's a doll" and then "give me a doll" she addresses the speech to a child, and then

> a child starts using its own language by saying 'A doll' and tries to grasp it. This is how, Luria says, "*the function, formerly divided between two*

*persons, becomes now a new form of an inner, self-regulated psychological process.*

(p. 4, Luria's emphasis)

In this text Luria spends most of the time discussing the role of speech and shows how in experimental settings children develop control over their motor actions through verbal commands. Also, he emphasizes the importance of seeing a brain as a whole, rather than studying its divided parts/functions, and suggests seeing it as a complex functional system. This is something that characterizes Luria's approach to the human – it is monistic in nature. His belief in the ability of 'monistic psychology' to hold to the 'dialectic of the whole organism' was already expressed in his article titled 'Psychoanalysis as a System of Monistic Psychology' in 1925 (Luria, 1977) and continued to be influential on his approach also when dealing with brain injuries. With the use of the functional system theory in clinical practice, he demonstrated how the restoration of lost functions was possible through compensation and reorganization of nervous connections. Luria's texts *Restoration of Function after Brain Injury* (1963) and *Traumatic Aphasia* (1970) illustrate this approach and present successful results of restorations after brain damage, including the restoration of the sense of self. It is important to note that Luria's approach to aphasia departs from the localization of damages and his understanding and classification of aphasia are based on the same principles as proposed by Freud in 1891. This indicates that Luria's later texts still should be read alongside Freud, despite the assumption that their theoretical grounds had moved apart.[15]

Nikolaeva (2011) suggests that Zeigarnik was a consistent follower of Vygotsky-Luria-Leontievian psychology. So we see that her understanding of the psychological meaning of the pathopsychological phenomena was based on their ideas regarding the function of the mind. The role of language as a symbolic mediator for the psyche, the close connection between affect and thinking, and the social-historical construction of the individual came from Vygotsky. Functional systems of the mind and departure from the brain localization models, and also memory as an active psychic function derived from Luria. The role of motivation in constructing symptoms, a hierarchy of motives and personality was taken from Leontiev.

### Zeigarnik's later career

In 1943 Zeigarnik became the head of the experimental pathopsychology laboratory at the Institute of Psychiatry in Moscow. In 1949 she began to teach courses on pathopsychology at Moscow State University. In 1950, however, she was suspended from her position at the Institute of Psychiatry and in 1953 dismissed. The reason for that was the Soviet anti-Semitic campaign of 1948–1953, or the Doctors' Plot; Rootless Cosmopolitan Campaign (Zeigarnik, 2001). For Zeigarnik, the 'thaw' (*ottepel*) happened only in 1957 when she was rehabilitated in her position at the Institute of Psychiatry. It is easy to underestimate to what extent antisemitism was present in the Soviet Russian society, and to estimate to what extent the hardship of life for Jewish scientists, like Zeigarnik, Luria and Bassin, contributed to the vicissitudes of psychoanalysis by redirecting their scientific interests into more safe areas or critical stances. We can estimate that a decent degree of freedom of thought was preserved by all of them, despite the dangers they had to endure.

In 1958, Zeigarnik completed her third doctoral dissertation, was granted a Doctor of Pedagogical Sciences degree and published her monograph, *Disturbances of Thinking in Psychiatric Patients* [*Narusheniia Myshleniia Psikhicheskikh Bol'nykh*] and, in 1962, her second monograph *Pathology of Thinking* [*Patologiia Myshleniia*]. It can be argued that the study of thought disorders was her main scientific interest. In her monographs, her extensive knowledge of the state of psychology and psychiatry, both Soviet and Western, strikes the reader. Still, Zeigarnik lived in the Soviet Union and freedom of thought was officially limited. References to Marx and Lenin were mandatory as was an obligation to criticize Western ideas for being 'bourgeois' and misplaced, so her writings had to address Western ideas carefully. In this time of relative freedom, Zeigarnik returned to her main interest – the study of thinking processes, and the expressions of thought disturbances in speech. Her extensive work on the question of schizophrenia gave rise to alternative ways of treatment and the social rehabilitation of patients.

The gradual turn away from Pavlov in Soviet science after the All-Union Conference on Philosophical Issues in the Physiology of Higher Nervous Activity and Psychology in 1962 allowed the return of psychology and the use of various methods in psychological research. In her later work, Zeigarnik evidenced psychologists' true attitude to Pavlov:

> The resolution [of that session] noted that, after the 1950 session, "the wide dissemination of a negative attitude toward psychology entailed practical harm and methodological error as some scholars tried to reduce the subject matter of psychology to the physiology of higher nervous activity.
> (Zeigarnik, 1973, pp. 14–15).

In 1965, she received the title Professor of Psychology and in 1967 was elected Chair of the Faculty of Psychophysiology and Neuropsychology at Moscow State University. In the following years she published several monographs: *Introduction to Pathopsychology* [*Vvedeniie v Patopsikhologiiu*] (1969), *Personality and Pathology of Activity* [*Lichnost' i Patologiia Deiatel'nosti*] (1971) and *Foundations of Psychopathology* [*Osnovy Patopsikhologii*] (1973, 1976). Together with Luria, in 1969 Zeigarnik attended the XIX International Congress of Psychology in London and chaired the session on experimental studies in abnormal psychology. In a way, Zeigarnik and Luria always shared views on the intimate connection nature of conscious activity with language. In 1972 her monograph on pathopsychology was published under the title *Experimental Abnormal Psychology* in English in New York and London (Zeigarnik, 1972).

Her life-long interest in the study of mind resulted in Zeigarnik's participation in the International Symposium on the Unconscious in Tbilisi in 1979. Years later, Zeigarnik co-authored a review of the Symposium in the journal *Voprosy Psikhologii*, titled 'The Problem of the Unconscious: Move to a Dialogue':

> The very existence of the symposium once and for all put an end to such myths that Western science was somehow inferior to Soviet science. It also marked the end of the harsh veto that allegedly existed in Russia.
> (Zeigarnik et al., 1987, p. 163).

The years before Zeigarnik's death aged 87 in 1988 proved fruitful. She gained international recognition for her work again, winning prizes in Germany and at home, and published multiple monographs that became classic handbooks for psychology students: *The Theory of Personality of K. Lewin* (1981) and *Theories of Personality in Foreign Psychology* (1982) and a new edition of her main work *Pathopsychology* (1986). In these monographs Zeigarnik shows deep understanding and knowledge of the history of the development of schools, from classic psychoanalysis to neo- Freudians, humanistic and existential psychology.

## *Zeigarnik reads Freud*

The way Zeigarnik discusses Freud's ideas, as we will see, calls into question her supposed critical attitude towards him.

Zeigarnik acknowledged that Freud had suggested the complexity and multidimensional nature of the structure of human behaviour. Her critique is directed against the opposition Freud places between the conscious and the unconscious. She read this as an antagonism between the individual and the social. Following Bassin, she accused Freud of a failure to include the social-historical dimension in his thinking, and for a correspondingly excessive biologization of behaviour through the notion of the Id and its impulses (Zeigarnik, 1982, p. 7). In line with Vygotsky who, as Zeigarnik points out, saw the future as one of the factors in the construction of behaviour, Freud is too focused on the past. This looks like a reiteration of the technique used by Bassin.

References to Freud appear in all of her main monographs (1958, 1962, 1981, 1982, 1986). Interestingly enough, Zeigarnik discusses Freud even in *The Theory of Personality of Kurt Lewin* [*Teoriia Lichnosti Kurta Levina*], the book which was supposed to be dedicated fully to Lewin's theory and to introduce the reader to its main concepts. This work includes extensive argument on the differences between the theories of Freud and Lewin, and it is clear that Zeigarnik held a deep knowledge of Freud's work. Zeigarnik mentions almost all the main Freudian ideas on: (1) the nature of the psyche; (2) personality; and (3) behaviour. Such a comparison of these two authors would not be possible without solid knowledge of both theories. Although the monograph was only published in 1981, it was formed from her lectures delivered at the Moscow State University from 1953 onwards and it meant that Zeigarnik had lectured about Freud's theory since the immediate post-Stalin years.

As a reader unfamiliar with the style of Soviet writings, one may question the necessity of such a mention of Freud in the text at all. As a reader looking at Soviet writings in the context of the socio-historical circumstances, one may assume that it was the only way for Freud to appear in the publication.

In the monograph *Pathopsychology [Patopsikhologiia]*, published in 1986, Zeigarnik gradually builds her approach to the study of the personality.[16] This was the second edition of her monograph on pathopsychology, with *Introduction to Pathopsychology [Vvedeniie v Patopsikhologiiu]* first being published in 1969. In the chapter introducing the pathopsychological experiment and ways of exploration of the personality she writes:

> The situation of the experiment included in itself everything from the theories of the other schools: ... the revival of associations, dreams, fantasies (Freud) etc. This form of experiment is not only the way to study phenomena, but also to create real situations. The pathopsychological experiment is designed precisely the same way.
> (Zeigarnik, 1986, p. 85)

According to this piece, the psychoanalytic approach to the study of associations, dreams and fantasies might be considered as a ground for her pathopsychological experiment. On the same page, without criticism, Freud's name appears when she introduces the basis for the methods of the study of the personality. She writes:

> When Freud applied his method of interpretation of dreams and slips of the tongue, he did it because he believed that human experiences are determined by unconscious powers, which are opposite to the conscious and thus they should reveal themselves in symbols.
> (Zeigarnik, 1986, p. 85)

Freud's appearance here is sudden, and references to him do not seem to be connected with the rest of the material in this chapter. It might, therefore, be reasonable to read this as an introduction to Freud, though a very brief one, rather than, or as well as, an overt criticism of him. This introduction is crucial if linked to her study of symbols in the speech of patients with schizophrenia.

However, it is less the direct references to Freud that indicate connections between Zeigarnik and psychoanalysis. Rather, it is her ideas on schizophrenia and her overall position towards mental disturbances expressed in her method of pathopsychology. Although Zeigarnik's main theoretical focus did not change much over the years, the pattern of her publications coincides with changes in science that were outlined in the previous chapter.

## The Soviet turn to biology: Schizophrenization of the country

It was not only the 1936 VKP(b) resolution 'On Pedological Perversions' that caused setbacks for Zeigarnik and Vygotsky and subjected their work to ideological obstruction.[17] The first years of Stalin's rule brought the first wave of biologization. Theories containing social and psychological reasoning were out of favour and official ideology proclaimed a Pavlovian turn to physiology (Krementsov, 1996, p. 260; Pollock, 2006, p. 104). Psychoanalysis could no longer provide the ground for understanding mental disorders.

Within the first few years of Stalin's rule, it became difficult for any Soviet psychologist to develop a psychosocial approach to research due to the country's ideological-political constraints. In the study of the relations between the political regime and psychiatry, Benjamin Zajicek argues that the term 'schizophrenia' was not in use in Soviet psychiatry during the 1920s. Ten years later, the situation had changed dramatically.

> During the 1930s, some psychiatric hospitals in the USSR were diagnosing 80 percent of their patients with schizophrenia, while at the same time claiming that up to 60 percent of schizophrenics remained undetected, living and working in the community.
> (Zajicek, 2014, pp. 167–168)

At first, Soviet psychiatry became oriented around so-called psychohygiene. This approach to social care regarding mental illness aimed at preventing mental illness from developing. Zajicek writes that in 1920 the government supported preventive medicine, but in 1930 psychiatrists lost the support of the Stalinist system, and a preventive approach was highly criticized: "the Commissariat of Public Health began to shift away from social hygiene and preventative medicine and toward a medical system that prioritized the needs of heavy industry" (Zajicek, 2014, p. 180). The shift from social reasoning and preventive medicine to physiological reasoning and treatment resulted in didactic orders from the party. "Schizophrenia – particularly in its 'acute and early forms' – was singled out as an example of the concrete disease entities that required increased concern" (p. 181).

The dream of a socialist society was not adequately realized for most people. To deal with the 'nervousness' of workers, the psychiatric system aimed to have control over citizens. The 'schizophrenia' diagnosis became widely overused by the Party to control dissatisfaction, tiredness and cases of evasion from work. New types, such as 'mild schizophrenia', appeared in the psychiatric arsenal, while criteria for diagnosis were vague:

> Sufferers were described as withdrawn or asocial, they had feelings of 'sluggishness,' 'apathy,' 'depression,' and irritability, and experienced odd bodily pains and 'neurotic reactions.' In the past, they had often been diagnosed as suffering from neurasthenia or exhaustion.
> (Zajicek, 2014, p. 186).

Accordingly, misuse of a 'schizophrenia' diagnosis illustrated the attempt by the Party to use psychiatric language to pathologize those members of the community who were not fulfilling their required role in society. More diagnostic subdivisions were created in the 1960s, when collaboration between some psychiatrists and party leaders resulted in the widespread practice of forced hospitalization of political dissidents and those who expressed different views to the main ideology (Zajicek, 2018). Another sub-category of schizophrenia emerged, "'sluggish schizophrenia', [vialo-tekushchaia shizofreniia], an allegedly profound mental illness that was also extremely difficult to differentiate from 'normal' states of mental health" (Zajicek, 2014, p. 167).

Abuse in psychiatry continued to exist throughout the future years of the USSR and cast a huge shadow on overall Soviet psychiatry in the West, as well as on public opinion of mental health practitioners. Such a reputation was also harmful for those workers in psychiatry and psychology who stayed away from the abuse and avoided collaboration with the Party.

### *Zeigarnik's alternative route*

Between 1936 and 1940, Bluma Zeigarnik did not publish any work, and until 1955 she did not publish anything on the question of disturbances of thinking and schizophrenia. It is curious that Zeigarnik did not contribute to the field during this period, in which the concept of schizophrenia received such significant attention. The reason for this can be found in understanding the differences between Zeigarnik's methods of diagnosis and the official psychiatric approach. Being largely divorced from biological reasoning, Zeigarnik's method of pathopsychology is based on an analysis of the patient's speech and their use of language. For instance, her first publication in the Soviet Union was titled 'To the problem of understanding the figurative meaning of words or sentences in pathological changes in thinking. Novel studies on apraxia, agnosia and aphasia' (1934).

Further work on disturbances of thinking, and especially those characteristics of schizophrenia, were summarized by Zeigarnik in two monographs: *Disturbances of Thinking of Psychiatric Patients* [*Narushenie Myshleniia u Psihicheski Bbol'nykh*] (1958) and *The Pathology of Thinking* [*Patologiia*

*Myshleniia*] (1962, 1965 in English). Despite the experimental language oriented to study individuals in their complexity, these monographs hold to ideas which were very close to Luria and Vygotsky. As we will see from the list of methods Zeigarnik used in her clinical work, she was focused on thinking, meaning that for her the most important criteria for diagnosis were neither an evaluation of symptoms nor success in completing tasks, nor personal traits. She was focused on understanding how the person's mind operates, following tracks of Vygotsky's 'semic method' and similar to psychoanalysis, how the thinking process structures the being in relation to the reality principle (Freud, 1911).

Even though at first glance it looks like a set of simple tasks, Zeigarnik's methods are designed to target areas that normally would not reveal themselves in the conversation between a psychiatrist and a patient. Zeigarnik mentions many times that some of the thought disturbances would never be apparent for colleagues or the family of a patient. However, it is important for a clinician to reveal these specifics in order to be able to diagnose correctly. Performed in a free order, these tasks structure the methodology of the diagnostic procedure called the 'pathopsychological experiment'.

The first method is *Variations of the associative experiment*. The aim of this task is to reveal the focus of the associations of the patient and the richness of connections with the previous experience presented in the verbal reactions (1958, 1965). The roots of the associative experiment she attributes to the work of Sechenov and the tradition of Russian psychiatry, but a reference to Jung and psychoanalysis is also present. The associative experiment was frequently used by the young Alexander Luria, who measured the emotional reactions of students and criminals (Proctor, 2020) and it might not be coincidental that it became one of Zeigarnik's research methods. However, in a way she is more psychoanalytic, as her accent is on the verbal reactions rather than physiological ones. The importance of verbal associations derives from her theoretical understanding of the mind (1956, 1965).

For Zeigarnik the meaning of the word occupies central place in regulating intellectual processes and higher psychological functions (1934). The key element for identifying disturbances of thinking processes to Zeigarnik is the distortion of the meaning of words. To be able to use words one should not only operate within the concrete meaning of the word, but also be able to include their broader sense and be flexible in using words outside their concrete meanings (1934, p. 133). This includes the use of metaphors and using words playfully. This is why another core task of the diagnostic procedure was *Explaining proverbs and metaphors, matching phrases and proverbs*. It explores an understanding of metaphorical meaning and abstract thinking (1956, 1965).

To be diagnosed with schizophrenia, a patient should show significant changes in their perception of the meaning of words: their use of language and their thinking process must change in very specific ways, when the language no longer serves as the function of connection with reality. Zeigarnik noticed that in schizophrenia distraction from the concrete meaning of words produces an endless flow of shifts of meanings, confusing the patient even more (1934, p. 99). For Zeigarnik this constitutes the major sign of schizophrenia.[18] Paradoxically, this charges words with extra meaning as the slippage is "caused less by a disturbance of concepts than by a tendency to classify any and every insignificant phenomenon as a particular 'concept'" (1934, p. 103). Every word becomes important for a patient and charged with meaning; the kind of investment described by Freud in the case of the Wolf Man (Freud, 1918). We see a great similarity to the understanding of schizophrenia in *The Unconscious* (1915), where Freud emphasizes that words are treated in schizophrenia as if they were objects and concrete things as though they were abstract (Freud, 1915, p. 203).

Invented by Luria, another task called *The method of pictograms* became a permanent part of Zeigarnik's methodology and proved to be sensitive to the changes in characteristics in thinking amongst patients with psychosis. It explores the process of memorization via the use of drawings – the task illustrates the symbolization processes of the patient. In a way, to be able to memorize given words and phrases via drawings, a patient must create their own symbols or rely on existing ones in the surrounding culture. That requires a certain ability for abstraction, as well as the subjective freedom to choose symbols independently. Results might also show the capacity to use metaphors (1958, 1965). This is how the psychotic structure reveals itself: quite often in this transition to the image, an acoustic form becomes the criterion for the creation of the pictographic image. Therefore, the symbol that a patient will use to memorize a given word of a phrase will not be a symbol in a strict sense, because it is not related to the word's meaning. The relationship between a word and its pictogram will be specific to the patient's own logic. And this, again, corresponds to Freud's idea of a distorted relationship between word presentations and object presentations in schizophrenia (1915, p. 196).

While the operation of thinking is formed by language and use of words, the origin of thinking for Zeigarnik is based in drives:

> Real human thinking (that which reflects the outside world) undoubtedly depends on human wants; intellectual activity, like any other human activity, is always directed towards the satisfaction of needs and always dependent on one's desires and feelings.
> It is, in fact, with the satisfaction of needs that the intellectual activity of man begins. This activity is at first purely practical (perceptual), and only later becomes theoretical.
>
> (Zeigarnik, 1965, p. 19)

She adds that, whereas the desire for the satisfaction of needs leads to the development of cognition and the attempt at objective reflection of the outside world, the same desires and needs might distort the course of thought and lead to cognitive errors (p. 19).[19] Such a definition of thought matches that given by Freud (1911) who sees it as "essentially an experimental kind of acting, accompanied by displacement of relatively small quantities of cathexis together with less expenditure (discharge) of them" (p. 220) where there is some "restraint upon motor discharge" (p. 220) of the drive. Ultimately, thinking is a substitute for action towards realization of the drive; initially unconscious it only later becomes "bound to verbal residues" (p. 220) and perceptible to consciousness. Neurotic and psychotic thinking is disturbed by the subject's wishes and aims to replace the disagreeable reality with the world of phantasy (Freud, 1924, p. 187).[20]

The desiring or motivational component of thinking in Zeigarnik's terms are explored in the pathopsychological diagnostic procedure as well. Invented by Vygotsky, the *Classification of objects* allows exploring the ways that the patient conceptualizes objects. Fluctuations of ideas produce constant shifts in meanings, which does not allow for a patient to 'stick' to certain categories; the conceptual field will be constantly moving, and a patient would not be able to create classifications for objects. Due to the affective response to certain categories, the patient will not be able to abstract and generalize objects into bigger groups. For example, to put the cat and the dog together as 'pet animals' might be impossible for the patient who doesn't like cats, therefore does not want them to be a pet.

A similar task, the *Exclusion of objects*, enables one to see how the generalization process works, and which elements become key for a patient, allowing one to link objects into the same group. It can be impossible for patients to exclude objects due to the affective link to certain concepts. In both of these tasks we see how the link between the affective component and thinking plays an important role in the diagnostic outcome.

Apart from the changes in thinking presented in the distortion of the usage of words, Zeigarnik found several more changes in thinking, specific to schizophrenia. These are changes in the logical course of thinking and disturbances of the purposiveness of thinking (1965, p.105; p. 149).[21] These changes would not be found in the case of fatigued citizens or by individuals who simply became distressed by the rigours of Soviet life. Accordingly, Zeigarnik's approach to diagnosis, which was more rigorous than the approved approach and excluded a vast number of citizens who had been pathologized by the State for their non-Soviet behaviour, was not useful for political manipulation.

Interestingly enough, during Brezhnev's rule between 1964 and 1982, when Soviet psychiatry re-entered an era of abuse, the 'sluggish schizophrenia' diagnosis was once again used by the Party to control dissidents. In that period, Zeigarnik's publications are more concerned with the role of personality in mental disturbances, emotional development, disturbances of thought processes, aphasia and the psychological consequences of brain damage. She discusses the role of pathopsychology in the system of mental care. Yet, once again, she does not mention schizophrenia. Only after 1985 would several of her publications on schizophrenia and hysteria appear in the *Korsakov Journal*.

Out of Zeigarnik's study of thinking, a new discipline crystallized in the mid-1960s – pathopsychology.

## The main principles of pathopsychology

Pathopsychology is a branch of psychology concerned with the study of changes in mental processes in mental disorders. Through an analysis of changes in perception, thinking, memory, and consciousness, it aims to also see general changes in the personality of the patient occurring with the disorder. Pathopsychology conceptualizes mental disturbances as alternative ways of organising mental processes, and on the basis of this decides on the category of the disorder. At the core of Zeigarnik's focus were changes in thinking, and it was crucial to differentiate between specific types of disturbances of thinking to differentiate between organic damage, psychoses and neuroses. Within psychoses she described specific changes in thinking, attributed to schizophrenia, that would not be found in delusional psychosis or other types of disorder.

Within the psychiatric system, pathopsychology belongs to the field of clinical psychology. The role of the clinical psychology within the psychiatric clinic was at that time to study mental disturbances in order to deepen clinical understanding of the genesis and prognosis of it (Zeigarnik, 1969). Even though clinical psychological laboratories within the psychiatric hospital existed, and in Saint-Petersburg was linked, for example, to the clinic founded by V. M. Bekhterev and in Moscow by S. S. Korsakov, they were less systemic. The big centre for the clinical psychology was also in the early 1930s in Kharkiv, Ukrainian SSR, where for several years Vygotsky worked on the theory and clinic of schizophrenia (Zeigarnik, 1969, p. 465).[22] In collaboration with Vygotsky and Luria, Zeigarnik created a system – a set of methods – that was reproduced in many clinics, at first in Moscow, and then more widely within Soviet Russia.[23] That establishment was very important for the psychiatric system, however it had to justify its methodology in the complex relationships with psychiatry, which was in 1950s inflamed by the Pavlov doctrine, when it came to the theory, and psychopharmacology, when it came to the treatment.

Zeigarnik emphasizes that the role of pathopsychology is to *describe* mental changes, to *understand the structure* of disturbed mental processes and to *relate it* to major psychiatric categories. Accordingly, I prefer not to use the English translation 'abnormal psychology' chosen in 1972 when Zeigarnik's monograph was published in the US. Zeigarnik suggests that what interests pathopsychology is to understand what is going on within the mind of a person, rather than to diagnose a person as 'abnormal' or suffering from a specific disorder. To give an explanation, and not establish a fact; it must explain the cause and source of reasoning of human behaviour, or some of the psychic phenomena[24] ... and aimed not at the study and measurement of the separate mental processes, but at the study of the human in his activity[25] [*deiatel'nost'*].

(Zeigarnik, 1986, p. 41, p. 43)

The diagnostic procedure according to the principles of pathopsychology is called the pathopsychological experiment. It is similar to a clinical interview, with some modifications – the main one being the use of specific methods, set tasks, discussed in the previous section of this chapter, to promote the conversation. Zeigarnik constructed the experiment in a way that provides the space for subjects to speak about their experiences, and not for the psychologist to evaluate the experience of the patient according to 'objective' standards, as, for example, in the Diagnostic and Statistical Manual. "Pathopsychological research reveals the real layer of life of the patient. That's why the programme of research on the patient in psychiatric practice cannot be fundamentally uniform and standardised" (pp. 53–54).

Each next step of the procedure depends on the outcome of the previous task. "The situation of the experiment should be structured like a chess game" (p. 84). The pathopsychologist should decide whether to proceed or not, and what direction to follow next, depending on what information was gained from the preceding conversation: "the experiment is intended to analyse the individual, not the features of their personality" (p. 86). Thus, the patient and the psychologist are in constant conversation. Together they are exploring the patient, analysing possible reasons for disturbance in the patient's life, much like patient and psychoanalyst, although in the different setting.

Zeigarnik argues that

> 'diagnostic' questions like: 'When are you in a better mood, in the evening, or in the morning?' should not be asked during the interview. Instead, if the patient says, 'I always feel bad, I don't want to do this, I don't want to do anything at all', it is better to ask 'Do you always do nothing? And how are you spending your time then? What are you doing?'

(p. 54).

This provides space for the patient to talk about his subjective experience.

"This approach is based on the right understanding of the causality of the mental activity, ... external conditions do not define activity and actions, and reason acts through 'internal conditions'", writes Zeigarnik (p. 45). We can see that the priority for pathopsychologists is internal reality, or psychic reality and internal reasoning, for the current condition of the patient. As a consequence, "pathopsychologists frequently face the accusation that their methods are not standardised but are subjective" (p. 53). The real aim of the experiment is to study the subject and explain the condition, based on an analysis of their psychic activity.

Another important part of the 'experimental' procedure is the analysis of 'mistakes' – any spontaneous answers given by patients 'without thinking', which are later corrected by patients themselves or by the experimenter. Mistakes often appear as meaningless answers; however, similarly to the Freudian approach to slips of the tongue and mistakes in action – which demonstrate the patient's unconscious content more than any of the subject's more conscious, directed thought – Zeigarnik considered mistakes as "the most interesting" source of knowledge about the patient, providing "material for assessing the disturbances of the mental activity of the patients" (p. 44). Zeigarnik introduces Freud's method in a different chapter of the same monograph; mentions of interpretations of dreams and slips of the tongue come later on page 82, which, again, does not seem to be accidental. Apart from tasks, pathopsychologists should pay attention to, and pick up details of, the reactions of the patient, that is, their emotional response. It is clear that Zeigarnik's approach is idiographic, analysing peculiarities and complexities.

After an experiment has finished, Zeigarnik suggests continuing the conversation with elements of psychotherapy, which she calls 'psychocorrection':

> The most important aspect of this conversation is to show the patient that it is not only the doctor or medications, but also him and his attitude, his action and his collaboration that helps the treatment procedure.
> (p. 60)

Even though the 'experiment' is concerned with studying perception, thinking and memory, Zeigarnik does not aim to study mental processes as biological events in the nervous system. Changes of the personality in her view are inevitably connected with changes of the core values, attitudes of the society and intentions of the person and his self- esteem; they are connected, although not in the linear, but more complex and mediated dependency with disturbances of the central nervous system. In analysis of these disturbances there is a danger of the mixture of psychological and biological categories. This mixture inevitably leads to covert, and thus the most dangerous, tendencies to explain psychological and social phenomena by biological causes. This slippage of psychological studies to the direct comparison of anatomical damages with behaviour changes may lead to the loss of the subject of the psychological research itself (p. 78).

Zeigarnik's extensive work on the question of schizophrenia gave rise to alternative ways of treatment and the social rehabilitation of patients. "Whereas general psychology investigates the regulating role of speech in the formation of voluntary movements, psychopathology shows the forms of disintegration of skilled movements resulting from the weakening of the regulating role of speech" (1965, p. 4). The concept of self-regulation became very important for Zeigarnik's later theory; we can summarize that the self-regulation achieved was via regulation through speech.

Zeigarnik was pointing out the need to create a special pathopsychological syndrome, where the understanding of the disturbance comes not from its phenomenological similarity, but is considered in relation to the core mechanism of its genesis. As Nikolaeva (2003) illustrates, further work of Zeigarnik's colleagues and disciples shows that such phenomenologically different states as anorexia nervosa and alcoholic addiction share the same psychological mechanism in their genesis. For psychoanalysts such logic does not appear as a discovery.

One of her last papers, written together with her disciples, was presented at the Symposuim on the Unconscious in Tbilisi in 1979 as 'The Attitude to One's Illness as a Condition for the Emergence of Conscious and Unconscious Motives of Activity'. In the paper, Zeigarnik and her co-authors studied patients' attitudes to their illnesses and their hypochondriac reactions. The authors argued for the importance of a disease's internal dynamics,[26] which influences a patient's emotional reaction towards the illness and affects the process of recovery. In other words, fantasies about illness produce changes in the condition of the patient. An important point here is that changes in the condition lead to personality changes and vice versa (Zeigarnik, Bakanova, Nikolaeva, and Sheftelevich, 1978). Again, we see how Zeigarnik encouraged paying attention to the reality of the patient and concentrating on their reactions towards their own psychic state. She uses the concept of the 'internal dynamics of disease' – psychoanalytically speaking, the phantasy – and its unconscious impact on the development of the disturbance. This shows that she recognized the unconscious. The internalized picture of illness, the role of personality, and the motivation of the patient are the focus of the process of rehabilitation.

Psychoanalysis holds to a set of formulations regarding the unconscious, thinking, language and schizophrenia, which are specific to it and cannot be found in other schools of thought. These are:

1   an understanding of the unconscious as not just non-conscious, but a complex structure with its own logic of operation (Freud, 1915);
2   that there exists an intimate connection between the unconscious and language, where words – presentations – serve as the substrate for thinking. Language acquisition for Freud opens the question of psychic reality, which includes thinking and internal perceptions (Freud, 1985);
3   that thinking which escapes the reality principle Freud calls 'phantasying' (1911), through which internal reality can depart from the reality of the outside world. Psychosis for Freud is based on the conflict between the ego and the external world, where the ego creates a 'new world' in accordance with the 'id's wishful impulses' (1924);
4   in the case of schizophrenia this departure can be traced to the level of the patient's language (1915).

Zeigarnik's work follows through and brings clinical confirmation to these formulations in her work on schizophrenia and the elements of pathopsychology. This can be explained either by the phenomena of simultaneous invention or by the influence of psychoanalytic ideas on her in these particular areas. Considering the presence of Freud's name in Zeigarnik's writings we can assume that these confluences possibly came from her familiarity with Freud's ideas. The fact that her closer colleagues Vygotsky and Luria were enthusiasts of psychoanalysis and that their ideas became the basis for Zeigarnik's pathopsychology can advocate for a further indirect influence through them.

Moreover, in times of prohibition of the 'bourgeois idealistic psychology', the unnecessary appearance of Freud's name in Zeigarnik's texts raises a question about its purpose. Given that his appearance is accompanied by exactly this standard addition of being an 'idealistic bourgeois wrong' author and that there is no other sort of critique provided, it is possible the real purpose of this 'criticism' was something else.

While Zeigarnik's contemporaries like Bassin spent many years rehabilitating the unconscious in Soviet psychology, as evidence of which we find multiple publications on this topic, she is not known for having such an explicit agenda in her own texts.

However, her lectures about Freud, Jung and the neo-Freudians, that she read from the 1950s at Moscow State University, can possibly be seen to indicate such an agenda.[27] An anecdote, given by a former student, can support such a suggestion. Once after a lecture, this student asked Zeigarnik, at that time in her late 70s, why she, a well-known professor, wasted her time reading lectures about these 'obscurantists, Freud and Jung' (these are Zeigarnik's words). In response, a silence and a 'wise look' was given to the student, who 'only later understood why', when she discovered how much hardship Zeigarnik had been through and how secretive a person she was despite her very open appearance. I see that episode as witness to another example of inconsistency – between criticism of the 'obscurantists' and over 20 years of repetition of their work, phenomena that don't quite match together. Her support of supervisees who openly engaged with psychoanalytic ideas in their first monographs (Sokolova, 1976; Nikolaeva, 1987), is another inconsistency. It is surprising that, as someone with very strong views against psychoanalysis, Zeigarnik would agree to supervise such work.

In the course of the development of Soviet society, early followers of psychoanalysis and their disciples found a way to keep their scientific interests intact. This, however, caused several complications. Strictly speaking the resulting theories are not psychoanalytic, as they departed from the mainstream of the psychoanalytic debate. Rather, they are original theories, concerned with the main psychoanalytic issues: the unconscious, thinking, language, and the origin of neuroses and psychoses. Moreover, they are not only concerned with the mind, but consider the individual as a whole: a body with a mind. At the same time, they cannot be seen as fully independent from psychoanalytic discourse, as ignoring their psychoanalytic roots distorts the meaning of their theoretical and clinical findings. Such a distortion leads to oversimplification, and, as post-Soviet history has shown, an effective abandonment of Soviet theories as outdated, or a portrayal of them as isolationist.

Zeigarnik's life and career was forged in a difficult era of Soviet history, when science was put under political and ideological control. To write and research freely at that time was difficult. Nevertheless, Zeigarnik proceeded with her research in the tradition she inherited from her three main teachers: Lewin, Vygotsky and Luria. Her discoveries on the psyche were crucial for further development of clinical psychology and psychiatry in the Soviet Union and Russia. Her method of the pathopsychological experiment has been developed widely and is still used in the contemporary psychiatric system. More importantly, having been developed in times of repression and violation of human freedom, the pathopsychological experiment is saturated with respect and care for the individual. Zeigarnik's work shows that it was not the case that the entire psychiatric system in the Stalinist era was abusive and dismissive of the subjectivity of the patient.

## Notes

1 While working with Kurt Lewin in Berlin in 1927, Zeigarnik discovered and experimentally proved that unfinished tasks are better remembered than finished tasks. This phenomenon received her name.
2 For the detailed analysis see Yasnitsky, A., The archetype of Soviet psychology: From Stalinism of the 1930s to the "Stalinist science" of our days. In Yasnitsky and Van der Veer (2015).
3 Sources for this collected timeline are presented fragmentarily in the memoirs of Zeigarnik's grandson Andrei (2001), *Zapisnye Knizhki (Notebooks)* of Vygotsky (2017) by Zavershneva and Van der Veer, *Rossiiskie Psikhoanalitiki* (*Russian Psychoanalyts*) (2000) by Ovcharenko and *Istoriia psikhologii v litsakh. Personalii* (History of Psychology in Personalies) (2005) by Karpenko.
4 In the Russian version of the book, Etkind made a connection between this paper and Luria's ideas on aphasia, which is curiously absent in the English translation.
5 That is not to say Luria and Vygotsky were interested only in psychoanalysis.
6 *Pravda*, 1924, No. 225.
7 *Remembering Completed and Uncompleted Tasks [Handlungen Das Behalten Erledigter und Unerledigter]*.
8 For a discussion and critique of Luria's Uzbeki expedition see the recent book by Proctor (2020). Also see the chapter 'The Primitive' and Chapter 8. Did Uzbeks have illusions? in Yasnitsky and Van der Veer (2015).
9 The description of the semic method, polemics and differences of it with approaches of Piaget and Levy-Bruhl to thinking and speech see in the Chapter 18, The Semic Method, in Zavershneva and van der Veer (2018). The same attitude is reproduced in Zeigarnik (1972).
10 For a more detailed account on Luria's experiments see Proctor (2020).
11 A more detailed discussion of Luria and brain is offered in the next chapter.
12 As well as Bassin, whose name will become important in the further chapter for his revitalization of the discussion on the unconscious and Freud in late 1950s, and many other psychologists.
13 GARF, f. R4737, op. 2, 1509

14 Proceedings to the XIX International Congress of Psychology in London, accessed online www.marxists.org/archive/luria/works/1969/conscious-action.pdf
15 This connection between Freud and Luria is explored in Solms (2000).
16 It is necessary to note that the Soviet term 'personality' is, in fact, very close to the concept of the subject in psychoanalysis.
17 For an important discussion on the continuation of 'suppression' of Vygotsky's work in the following years see Fraser and Yasnitsky (2015). This raises the question of the extent to which the establishment of the 'Stalinist model' of psychology contributed to the omission of links with psychoanalytic theory.
18 An interesting parallel can be drawn between this understanding of schizophrenia and Lacanian notion of 'le point de capiton' and psychosis defined as a slippage in the chain of signifiers (Lacan, Seminar III).
19 Zeigarnik is critical of Bleuler, who isolates affective thinking from rational thinking; for her, this is an impossible division as thinking is always related to the affective reaction.
20 For altered thinking Freud elsewhere uses a term *phantasying* (Freud, 1911, p. 222).
21 This departs from the theoretical understanding of thinking in Gestalt psychology, which was insufficient for Zeigarnik, not only "as objects outside of consciousness did not exist for the Gestalt psychologists" (1972, p. 49) and because "the process of thinking is reduced ... to an equilibrium between dynamic forces and fields. Neither past experience, nor acquired knowledge, nor speech plays a significant role in thinking. Thinking is detached from the outside world and from human practical activity. The qualitative features of human thought processes are eliminated" (1965, p. 22) and "as Vygotsky so clearly expresses it, in Gestalt psychology there is no line of demarcation in principle between human mental activity and the behaviour of the earthworm" (p. 22). As Vygotsky highlights, Zeigarnik and Birenbaum's study of thinking (1934) departs as well from Lewin's understanding of thinking in the theory of field (Zavershneva and van der Veer, 2018, p. 334–336, p. 410).
22 To remind the reader that Bassin originally worked in Kharkiv before moving to Moscow, and Luria spent several years there as a head of the laboratory of psychology.
23 A school of Zeigarnik is still strong nowadays in Russia, and pathopsychology is practiced by clinical psychologists widely in psychiatric hospitals and psychoneurological dispensaries.
24 Here and further references are given from Zeigarnik texts in Russian, in my own translation, except for references to the monograph *The Pathology of Thinking* (1965).
25 'Activity theory' is a term developed by Vygotsky, see Kozulin (2005).
26 The term 'internal dynamics [image] of disease' was invented by therapist Roman Luria (father of Alexander Luria) in 1935. It postulates the importance of the patient's subjective perception of the illness as it has an impact on the development of the illness and the success of the treatment. The internal picture of illness can be seen as the unconscious structure, including body image, self-perception, the idea of the disease. This dynamic structure has impact on the emotional responses of the patient towards illness, including the appearance of the secondary gain.
27 See memories of Leonora Pechnikova, 8:48:00 www.youtube.com/watch?v=y_MCnxOeUfU

Chapter 4

# Luria's turn to psychophysiology, language and consciousness

It is difficult to imagine the psychoanalytic movement in Soviet Russia without young Alexander Luria, whose effort and engagement in the activities of the Psychoanalytic Society were the key to its existence. As already mentioned, in 1921, he established the Psychoanalytic Society in Kazan. After his move to Moscow, he continued to participate in the scientific activity of the Russian Psychoanalytic Society by being its secretary until 1927, regularly presenting at its scientific meetings and giving lectures.

In many sources on the history of Soviet psychology and the psychoanalytic movement in Russia, however, it is claimed Luria abandoned his interest in psychoanalysis, which changed into an interest in neuropsychology and brain studies. His pupils would not recognize psychoanalysis as a valid theoretical contribution to Luria's work. For someone ingrained in psychoanalytic theory, however, Luria's turn to physiology was not marked by the departure from psychoanalysis, but the necessity of the historical kind. "His (ostensible) abandonment of psychoanalysis was undoubtedly the result of political and ideological pressure, rather than of developments in his scientific thinking" (Solms, 2000, p. 92). So that the similarities found by Solms between Luria's and Freud's thinking logically derive from an interest in psychoanalysis that was never lost.

In 1967, Italian psychoanalyst Cesare Musatti met Alexander Luria during a visit to the Soviet Union. Musatti noted that, of course, some reservations about practicing psychoanalysis under the socialist regime, as well as recognition of the challenges involved in organizing psychoanalytic activities, were expressed by members of the receiving group, (among whom was also Filipp Bassin). During that meeting, Luria showed Musatti a letter he had received from Freud in 1922, in which Freud addressed him as 'Sehr geehrter Herr Präsident'. The following curious episode tells us more about Luria's relationships with psychoanalysis in a Freudian way:

> After the meeting, while we were dressing ourselves to go outside, Luria accidentally put on my coat. Everyone laughed and agreed to interpret this failed act as an expression of an unconscious desire to 'be in my

DOI: 10.4324/9781003527268-5

This chapter has been made available under a CC-BY-ND 4.0 license.

shoes': to have continued to be a psychoanalyst in a country where psychoanalysis was permitted, continuing to be President of a Psychoanalytic Society, as I was in those years in Italy.

(Angelini, 1988, p. 13)

This chapter focuses on the shift in Alexander Luria's career from psychology to physiology, and how his research in neuropsychology and psychophysiology that developed from the 1930s interacted with ideas about the unconscious. It seeks to understand Luria's transition from psychologist to neuropsychologist and brain researcher, using the archival documents around the defence of his doctorate degree in psychology in Tbilisi and the transfer of it to Moscow in the late 1930s, arguing that the engagement with physiology was both forced and genuine for Luria. The set of archival documents examined in this chapter has not yet been discussed in the existing literature and is most likely presented here for the first time. In this chapter I also outline some of Luria's ideas on the role of language in the formation of the mind and will in addition, attempt a parallel reading of Luria's texts with psychoanalytic ideas.

## The search for a new science

Looking back at his career in his memoires, Luria wrote about his relations with scientific psychology and dissatisfaction with the academic psychology of that time.

> I also found academic psychology terribly unattractive because I could see no way to connect such research to anything outside the laboratory. I wanted a psychology that was relevant, that would give some substance to our discussions about building a new life.
>
> (Cole and Levitin, 2006, p. 22)

As we've seen in the previous chapters, psychoanalysis was one of the theories that offered Luria a promise about new ways of studying the mind. In the text 'Psychoanalysis as a System of Monistic Psychology' (1925) he highlights a systemic approach to the study of the mind that psychoanalysis offers: "Instead of studying discrete, isolated 'elements' of mental life, psychoanalysis attempts to study the whole personality, the whole individual, his behaviour, inner workings, and motive forces" (Luria, 1925, p. 14).

Already in 1925, the systemic study of the mind for Luria included the study of the body and nervous system:

> This, indeed, is the only way that psychology can, instead of taking the philosophical and metaphysical road toward constructing a monistic theory of personality, set out along the promising path of science toward mastering this problem, namely, by linking the specific motive forces of

the organism and its behaviour with processes taking place in the nervous system and the body's organs, and by ascertaining the role of these organs in psychoneural activity.

(Luria, 1925, p. 17)

The study of the body, nevertheless, does not exclude a psychoanalytic approach to it:

Despite the forced psychological terminology of psychoanalysis, which strikes the eye at first glance, it approaches the individuals as an integral organism, in which the anatomical structure and the functions of the individual organs, the drives, and higher mental activity are all integrally interrelated.

(Luria, 1925, p. 18)

Moreover, as my research attempts to demonstrate, Luria never truly attacked or abandoned his relations with psychoanalysis[1] and we must keep this in mind while reading his later works. He could not, at the same time, directly reference Freud. As we've discussed earlier, Luria was persecuted by the authorities for his interest in psychoanalysis. Even when The Russian Psychoanalytic Society was dissolved, and despite leaving the position of its secretary, Luria continued to receive disciplinary warnings for his engagement with Freud's ideas. That was for a reason:

Despite this pressure, Alexander Romanovich, who had plenty of reason to join in the renunciation of Freudian theory as a result of his own theoretical work, failed to engage in denunciations. Instead, he confined his references to psychoanalytic research to purely methodological and empirical points. For example, his development of the combined motor method, which dominated *The Nature of Human Conflicts*, was conceived as a kind of neo-Freudian experimental reconciliation of experimental-explanatory and clinical-descriptive approaches to the study of mind and emotion.[2] Although Freud and Jung are barely mentioned in the monograph, this fact is not an egregious slight but rather, considering the pressure to expunge them altogether, a stubborn insistence that the historical record not be completely obliterated.

(Cole and Levitin, 2006, p. 211)

Luria's publication in the *Internationale Zeitschrift für Psychoanalyse* titled 'Die moderne russische Physiologie und die Psychoanalyse' [The Modern Russian Physiology and Psychoanalysis] (1926) reflected his intent to fuse psychoanalysis and physiology. His early interest in experimental techniques combined with psychoanalysis was apparently described in a mystery article in English, titled 'Ways to Experimental Psychoanalysis' dated in the same year as an article by Luria that was published in the Psychoanalytic Review.[3] However, no trace of this publication in the PR archival issues was found.

Luria's studies of affective reactions which he conducted throughout the 1920s are known from the published work *The Nature of Human Conflicts* (1932 in English, 2002 in Russian). Already in there, Luria attempted to measure physiological responses while using psychoanalytic theory to explain it. In this combination, however, Luria was interested more in psychology rather than physiology of the phenomena he encountered. As noticed by Proctor (2020), even though he failed to provide a cultural-historical basis to explain the psychology of his experimental subjects, Luria succeeded in implementing a unified approach to the study of the body and mind.

From the beginning, Luria's intention was to find an explanation for psychological functions. And despite the fact that he was a founder of neuropsychology, his studies were far from only brain studies. The link between subject, psyche and brain was crucial for Luria.[4] Adolph Meyer would write about him, "Luria offers us a true psychobiology and not largely neologizing tautology" (Cole and Levitin, 2006, p. 36).

## Luria and the brain

Known as a father of neuropsychology in Russia, Luria indeed spent a huge part of his scientific career studying various effects of brain damage. Often compared with Oliver Sacks, Luria falls in the 'brain studies scientist' category, which by its very mention causes aversion in that part of psychoanalytic circles concerned with the talking cure method. Although neuropsychoanalysis is nowadays a growing field that could easily incorporate Luria's work – and, in fact, is doing so (Solms, 2000) – it is still unclear what Luria has to do with those psychoanalytic schools that keep language and relationships at the forefront, rather than the brain.

Homskaya, a former pupil of Luria who wrote his first full intellectual biography, insists on "Luria's contribution not only to neuropsychology, which is not in doubt, but also to other spheres of psychological science (general, historical, developmental psychology, defectology, and psychophysiology)" (2001, p. 114). This argument on the primary psychological interest of Luria is going to be my main thread for this discussion and will outline the place his research can occupy in the history and theory of psychoanalysis.

As we have seen in previous chapters, there is no doubt as to the early enthusiasm of Luria in engaging with psychoanalysis in the 1920s. The turning point, however, was the 1930s, when Luria 'changed his career' and finished medical school. Homskaya points out that Luria started to attend some of the medical classes from 1926, and Luria's daughter confirms that in 1937 he graduated from the First Moscow Medical Institute. However, she cannot say exactly why he decided to do that:

He couldn't help but see the threat that he is in trouble, especially since after the Central Asian expeditions he was already was on the verge of being arrested. And yet, it's not so easy to give up two well-run [psychological] laboratories, because of the need to graduate from medical school.

(Luria, 1994, p. 76)

Between 1926 and 1937 a lot of changes happened in Luria's life. He resigned as a secretary of the Psychoanalytic Society in 1927, went on psychological expeditions to Uzbekistan and Kirghizia, Central Asia in 1931–1932, worked in Kharkiv as a Head of the Section of Psychology at the Psychoneurological Academy of the Ukraine in 1931–1933 and went back to Moscow where he worked as the Head of the Department of Psychology at the Medico-Genetic Institute (also called the Moscow Medical Institute of Genetics) in 1933–1936. This biographical list shows that up to 1936, the year when pedology became outlawed, Luria kept his interest in psychology intact. After graduating from medical school, Luria became resident in the Institute of Neurosurgery, where he began to develop *psychological* methods of diagnosis of brain damage (Luria, 1994, p. 89). Again, psychology came first, even after the forced transition.

Some archival findings shed light on the turbulence Luria had experienced in the 1930s because of his interest in psychology. These are documents from the personal folder of Luria in GARF,[5] containing various documents around both of Luria's doctorate dissertations, in psychology and in medicine:

1   stenography of the meeting dedicated to the discussion of his doctorate thesis in Tbilisi, 05/01/1938;
2   several documents around Luria's application in Moscow to approve his degree, including the transcript of the expert commission in pedagogy meeting from 08/06/1939, the letter from Kornilov with the review of Luria's doctorate dissertation and his scientific work (uncertain/1939), the transcript of the Higher Attestation Commission, VAK on the approval of Luria's doctorate degree in psychology Moscow from 23/06/1939;
3   several documents around Luria's doctorate dissertation in medical sciences, including the transcript of the scientific meeting in Kyiv Medical University from 10/05/1943, several reviews on Luria's dissertation, the transcript of the VAK commission on the approval of Luria's doctorate degree in medicine Moscow from 10/06/1944.

From these documents it is clear that Luria had been persecuted for his connections with psychoanalysis up until 1939.

Apparently, Luria applied to defend his dissertation in psychology for the doctorate degree in pedagogical sciences in Tbilisi State University in 1938. That same year he applied for the degree to be approved by the Higher Attestation Commission (VAK) in Moscow.[6] The work was sent to Prof

Kornilov, at that time the Director of the State Psychology Institute, with the request for a review.[7] The letter from Kornilov is replete with doubts about Luria's academic rigour, especially when it comes to so-called 'mistakes', meaning that Luria is not trustworthy and still engaging with wrong theories, including Freud's ideas. As far as 1939, as we can see, Luria was deemed not free from his 'past mistakes'. It took the commission a year to decide and only in 1939 was he awarded the degree of the doctor of pedagogical sciences (in psychology).[8]

Let us look in more detail at the stenograph of the commission's meeting on the 8 July 1938.[9] After the long hearing, the commission did not come to an agreement, as three members voted 'for' and three 'against' awarding Luria the doctorate degree:

> The scientific and practical activity of Luria in the recent past was based on methodological foundations, essentially anti-Marxist, which contributed to the introduction of the pseudoscience of pedology into Soviet psychology and pedagogy.
> Presented work, defended by Luria A.R. for the degree of Doctor of Pedagogical Sciences, according to the reviews of comrades Kornilov and Georgiev, suffers from methodological errors, and in some places indicates that Luria is still largely in captivity of the anti-scientific cultural-historical theory, which did not allow him to complete his dissertation as a whole to put on a high theoretical level.[10]

The next VAK commission document from the archive is dated 8 June 1939.[11] Members present were Prof. Rubinstein, comrade Kornilov, Prof. Kolbanovskii,[12] Prof. Shimbelev,[13] comrade Plotnikov,[14] and Prof. Smirnov.[15] From this document we can get more detail about Kornilov's position towards Luria and details on the investigation of Luria's expedition to Central Asia and the publication of *The Nature of the Human Conflicts* in America. It also comes with the reference letter that Kornilov provided by the request of the commission, that caused a delay in Luria's award.

Let's look closer to what Kornilov says in this letter[16]:

> The review of the scientific and practical activities of A.R. Luria:
> I have known A.R. Luria since 1923, when he, as a junior researcher, began his work at the Institute of Psychology, where I was the Director at that time. With his youth, good training for scientific work (knowledge of languages, literature), A.R. Luria brought with him to the Institute an extreme passion for the teachings of Freud. Soon a whole *group of Freudian scientists (Luria, Vygotsky,*[17] *Zalkind, Reisner, etc.)* was formed at the Institute of Psychology. On this basis, I had numerous fundamental disagreements with A.R. Luria. This continued until 1926, approximately, when, in connection with the struggle against Freudism, raised in the

journal 'Under the Banner of Marxism', this enthusiasm for Freudism was eliminated. *The remnants of this Freudism are still preserved in the doctoral dissertation* of A. R. Luria.

In 1928–1929, A.R. Luria, together with Vygotsky, put forward the theory of the cultural-historical development of the psyche and published the book Cultural- Historical Essays, in which views alien to Marxism were developed. This theory of 'cultural-historical development' was finally exposed in the psychological discussion of 1931 as anti-Marxist.

In 1932 A.R. Luria, together with the American professor Koffka, undertook an expedition to Uzbekistan on behalf of the Institute of Psychology (the director at that time was Comrade Kolbanovskii) to study the thinking of the Uzbeks. As a result of this expedition, A.R. Luria and prof. Koffka revealed that the Uzbeks seem to have special forms of thinking, qualitatively sharply different from the ways of thinking of the common European peoples. The dissemination of this essentially racial theory of thought was put to an end by a survey carried out by the Institute of Psychology by the Moscow Committee of the Party, which qualified this theory as 'counter- revolutionary'. A.R. Luria had to leave his job at the Institute of Psychology and transferred his work to Kharkiv, where he simultaneously entered the medical faculty as a student.

For some time in the same years 1932–1935 A.R. Luria worked at the Moscow Genetic Institute, where he did research on twins. But, since the Genetic Institute was soon liquidated, as it carried out ideas alien to Marxism, the work of A.R. Luria ceased, being perceived as obviously ideologically unrestrained.

During this time, A.R. Luria drew up his research into a book, which he published in America in English. But even here, he makes gross mistakes of a purely political nature, in the form of an indication that 'purges' of students took place in Soviet universities, which gave him the [experimental] material for his research.

It is extremely characteristic that during all this time A.R. Luria never appeared in print, nor did he speak about criticizing his errors and mistakes. It would seem that the defence of a doctoral dissertation was a convenient opportunity for this, but here, too, A.R. Luria avoided defending this dissertation in Moscow and defended it in Tbilisi.

A year or two before A.R. Luria completed his medical education he began working at the Neurosurgical Institute. *But he did not stop working in the field of psychology,* and since March 1938, when he again became the Director of the Institute of Psychology, he was entrusted with the leadership of the pathopsychological section that had opened at the Institute. It would seem that numerous methodological errors should have taught A.R. Luria caution. It turned out not to be so: at the very first meeting of the section, where he made a report, A.R. Luria expounded, not only not critically, but with pathos, the linguistic theory of the phoneme of the White emigrant, the former Prince [Nikolay] Trubetzkoy.[18] Fortunately, the meeting was attended by Prof. Artemov, who rebuffed this theory and its speaker.

My final conclusion is such: A.R. Luria is a talented researcher in the sense of mastering the methods of experimental psychological research, but ideologically a completely intemperate person. You can never vouch for his report, speech, article, that it will not contain the grossest ideological errors and blunders. He can work perfectly under constant supervision and guidance, but he cannot be entrusted with an independent and responsible area of work, because in essence *the entire conscious life of this scientist is almost a continuous methodological error.*

Prof. Kornilov, director of the Institute of Psychology?/I-39 (January 1939)[19]

During the commission he repeated his position towards Luria:

> That is why I say that this particular work is quite worthy of a doctor if taken in isolation, and if you take the whole behaviour of a person, I believe that putting him in an independent responsible area where he can work without control – I would not do that, because he did not publicly declare his guilt anywhere.... To say that it arises from this that Luria is an anti-Soviet scientist is incorrect, but this is a person for whom I cannot vouch, and if you can vouch for it, that's your business.[20]

We can see that the attitude of Kornilov is quite harsh as he calls Luria's scientific life 'a methodological error' and emphasizes that he is not trustworthy as a person for his engagement with Freud, his mistakes in the Central Asian expedition and the publication of *The Nature of Human Conflicts* in America. Members of the commission had to undertake an investigation of the circumstances of all that was mentioned above. Apparently, they had a more supportive attitude towards Luria, and had to master their arguments to acquit Luria from his mistakes. Below is an account of what they came up with:

Regarding the Central Asian expedition,[21] the accusation that Luria's ideas are racist comes from the comparison of his observations on the different kinds of thinking presented by Uzbekipeople with "the racist theory of 'primitive' people[22] of Levy-Bruhl". This is a misunderstanding, points out Smirnov, as Luria relates the differences in thinking to socio-economic, and not to racial origin. Luria's interest in Freud is assigned to the mistake of 'youth'.[23] The publication of his dissertation in English is explained by delays. It was written in 1932–1933 and submitted for publication to the Uchpedgiz (Educational and Pedagogical State Publishing House) and simultaneously in agreement with the publisher was given for a translation to America. It was expected that due to the need to translate the work into English first, and then the usual editorial and publishing process, the work will be published in

America later. However, in Uchpedgiz work was subjected to multiple checks and Luria had to make substantial corrections, which he did and transformed this work into the doctoral thesis that he presented for defence in Tbilisi State University. This took three to four years, and meanwhile the work was published in America.[24] Thus, argues Smirnov, this is a mere coincidence.[25] Moreover, continues Smirnov, the fact that Luria's dissertation was already discussed five times by the VAK and the focus of the discussion is not on the quality of work and whether it deserves an award of the doctorate degree, but more on the reputation of Luria as a bourgeois and anti-Soviet scientist, turns the discussion into a socio-political matter. He concludes:

> We need to resolve the issue of Luria's academic degree and thus the burden that haunts him will be lifted. Now Luria is in such a position, that wherever he goes, legends, rumours, whispers, etc. always accompany him. Everywhere he has to explain that he had mistakes as he did this and that.[26]

The issue was resolved a month later, on 23 June 1939 at the final VAK commission, where the decision of the award was eventually made.[27] This time, it was a different set of members in the commission: Romanovskii,[28] Smirnov, Kolbanovskii, Kaftanov,[29] Gagarin.[30] Kornilov was not amongst them, and by the tone of their presentations it is apparent they were there to help Luria. In the opening speech, it was stated that a discussion around Luria's degree had already happened many times without success, predominantly due to the review given to his work by Kornilov. Smirnov noted that Luria had been investigated in the past in relation to his Central Asian expedition. A new investigation of his 'case' was made, and results were presented as such:

> The fact is that Comrade Luria made several mistakes in his previous works because he was a follower of Freud. Indeed, in 1925 he published in a journal edited by Prof. Kornilov an article in which there were major errors. At that moment he was only 24 years old.[31] We were interested in the question of how Comrade Luria now regards these mistakes and whether he himself criticizes his previous mistakes. We have established that in several later works, he criticizes his own work and the work of Freud in general, while he takes the completely correct positions of Marxist-Leninist methodology. Thus, Comrade Luria was mistaken, but these mistakes belong to his past.[32]

Furthermore, based on several facts from Luria's biography, Smirnov concluded that Luria had 'worked' on his mistakes. Firstly, Luria studied in Marx-Lenin University to fill the gap of his Marxist education. Secondly, Luria realized that to be a good physiologist[33] he needed to study anatomy and physiology. Therefore, he entered the Medical University and completed it perfectly well. Also, Luria was the head of the Psychology Department in the Institute of Psychology and a doctor in the neurosurgical institute. He was a talented scientist and published major articles in his field. Then, a further two very interesting facts were noted: "Luria was a follower of Vygotsky, who was a very talented person", and his dissertation was approved by big scientists in the University of Tbilisi, and "everyone knows that scientists of Tbilisi University are known experts in psychology, therefore we should not have any doubts"[34] in their decision.[35]

Another member of the commission, Gagarin, pointed out:

> A few days ago I had to talk to Comrade Luria and deal with his case.... The positive quality of Comrade Luria is that now he has realized that it is no longer possible to share Freudian mistakes and Freudian theory. He realized that a full-blooded Marxist psychologist has no right to share the Freudian point of view.[36]

Several moments in these few sentences are important to note. This took place in July 1939, meaning that it had been 12 years since Luria left the Psychoanalytic Society when the discussion around his affinity to Freudian theory took place. Linguistically, it is interesting, too, that 'Luria realized that it is no longer possible' and 'he has no right'. Gagarin could have said that Luria is no longer interested, or no longer shares Freud's views. In my view this summarizes neatly the situation Luria found himself in – the impossibility to do what he wanted to do, rather than a change of interest.

Now, what was the role of Kornilov in this trial? This time he was not invited to be present in person. It was discussed that he held an ambivalent position towards Luria's dissertation and work as a whole. On the one hand, he approved the dissertation which was sufficient enough for Luria to be awarded a doctorate degree. On the other hand, he emphasized that Luria made a lot of 'mistakes'[37] and does not deserve to be an independent scientist, and that in addition he needed supervision of his work because he will be most likely to repeat his 'mistakes' in the future.[38]

The final question that was discussed by this commission is to which discipline Luria's work belongs. Kolbanovskii suggested that Luria should be given the award of doctor of biological sciences, since his work is based on physiological experiments and therefore belongs to biology more than to pedagogy.[39] Overall, he argued, psychology should belong to biology, rather than to pedagogy. Gagarin, on the other hand, objected to such an allocation. Of course, the name of Pavlov came up in this discussion immediately. Kolbanovskii argued that the works of Pavlov are pure biology. Gagarin retorted that what Pavlov wrote about psychology deserves a lot of critique, and that a science about conditional reflexes is not a psychology.[40] Overall, it was decided to stay within pedagogy and Luria was awarded a degree as such.

It is important to note here that in the document from 10 October 1938 Luria's dissertation is titled "The Analysis of the Affective Processes" [K analizy affektivnosti processov],[41] while in 28/05/1942 in the document where the work is recommended for the publication, its title is mentioned as "Psychophysiology of Affective Processes" [Psikhofiziologiia affectivnykh processov].[42] Thus, the inclusion of biology, as Kolbanovskii insisted, eventually happened at least on the level of the title.

As we already know, during WWII, Luria worked in the town of Kisegach with a team of researchers, rehabilitating and studying brain injuries – the subject that was suitable for the time not only ideologically. There Luria collected the research material and on 19 May 1943 defended his dissertation in Kyiv Medical University. On 25 April 1944, his degree was approved in Moscow, and he received a doctorate in medical sciences and a professorship in neuropathology for his work on aphasia. The title of his dissertation was "Studies of Aphasia in the Light of Brain Pathology. Temporal Aphasia". A brief summary suggests that in that work Luria is interested in studying the phonology of aphasia, and a linguistic approach is included in his methods, which is an area that had never been studied before.[43]

In 1945, a new director of the State Institute of Psychology, S. R. Rubinstein, applied to the Higher Education Commission to appoint Luria (among several others) as a professor of psychology.[44] His request was declined "because Luria had already been granted a professorship in neuropathology".[45] That was another turn of events, that kept Luria's name apart from psychology and that contributed to the general perception of Luria as related predominantly to the neuro-sciences.

However, the trouble for Luria had not ended. In the 1950s Luria suffered from the consequences of the Pavlov Session: he was blamed for anti-Pavlov studies in psychology. Simultaneously Luria was a subject of attack by the campaign against cosmopolitanism (Doctor's Plot, or antisemitic campaign) (Homskaya, 2001):

> In 1951, the laboratory of Alexander Romanovich at the Institute of Neurosurgery of Burdenko was closed. Upset by this event, it seemed to Luria that he would never be able to return to his favourite work. To continue his activity, Luria transferred to the Institute of Defectology of the Academy of Pedagogical Sciences of the Russian Federation, directed by L. V. Zankov.
>
> (Homskaya, 2001, pp. 42–43)

This was not only a loss of the place for him to continue the work he loved. Overall, security of life was also taken from him again. Luria's daughter remembers her father being ready not to return from work and that he had a 'suitcase' packed in case of an arrest, during the years of the Doctor's Plot (Luria, 1994, p. 146).

Despite this, his interest in psychology persisted. Together with Leontiev, Luria founded the "first Psychology Department in the country" (Homskaya,

2001, p. 115) in Moscow University in 1966. Furthermore, Homskaya points out that "for Luria as well as for Vygotsky, psychology was an applied science, serving the interests of clinical practice" (p. 116). This was the time when Zeigarnik and colleagues actively promoted pathopsychological research, aimed at the study and support of mental health patients.

In the 1970s, Luria

> proclaimed that instead of the elementary psychological acts of the motor reaction type, the focus of research had to be shifted onto the complex conscious-cognitive forms of behaviour, such as a meaning-oriented perception and voluntary memory, solving intellectual problems, processing and previewing of behavioural situations and so on.
>
> (Homskaya, 2001, pp. 78–79)

For example, 'functional systems' (P. K. Anokhin) and 'physiology of activity' (N. A. Bernstein), "capable of explaining the self-determined and active character of human behaviour" (p. 79). These were not new ideas, however, as Luria had already mentioned the importance of the study of complexes and functional systems in 1930 (Hames, 2002).

What can we gain from a reading of these archival documents? Luria, at that time, was quite an established scientist in Moscow. He went to Tbilisi, Georgia to defend his dissertation in psychology and to Kyiv, Ukrainian SSR to defend his dissertation in medicine. 'Rumours and whispers' accompanied Luria for over ten years, from the late 1920s up to the 1940s for his 'mistakes', which included the affinity to Freud. Luria's 'turn to neuropsychology' and 'brain studies', as we see, was forced by the circumstances of that time, and his persistence in doing psychological research caused him a lot of trouble, including the danger of being accused of partaking in anti-Soviet activity. Luria, without doubt, was more than just a follower of psychoanalysis. He was aiming to enrich and transform existing methods and theories, combining multiple approaches together. Hence, it is a simplification to see him only as a 'father of neuropsychology' or as a brain scientist.

## Luria, language, consciousness, and Freud

If we take seriously that, as Bogdanchikov notices, "without the influence of psychoanalysis, all subsequent general psychological and neuropsychological constructions of A. R. Luria would not have been so carefully thoughtful and convincing – both for A. R. Luria himself, and for all scientific communities" (2002, p. 84), could it be that further studies that Luria conducted, in fact, might be nuancing some of Freud's ideas?

In this section of the chapter I will attempt a close reading of Luria's works on the question of the role of language in development of the mind. The aim of this reading is to discover potential links between Luria's work and Freud's work and more importantly, what Luria's studies have to offer to psychoanalysis, especially on the role of the language in the formation and functioning of the mind.

To start, I must first return to Zeigarnik and Vygotsky, whose work can explain with more clarity the concept of self-regulation and mediation. While Zeigarnik did not give a lot of credit to psychotherapy (or there is a general consensus that she didn't), she recognized the power of verbal exchange and its curative potential. It's often reiterated in her works that a good conversation between a pathopsychologist and a patient has the potential for improving a patient's mental state. The basis for this lies in the concept of self-regulation (*samoregulatsiia*). In short, self-regulation is the ability of the person to regulate their activity, emotions, and thinking through mediation.[46] While a healthy individual uses mediation in a way that it does not disturb activity, patients with mental health issues tend to concentrate excessively on mediation (Zeigarnik, 1972, pp. 41–41).

In the second edition of the *Pathopsychology*, published in the comparatively free year of 1986, the role of mediation is mentioned in relation to 'psychocorrection'. In the conversation during the pathopsychological experiment procedure, a psychologist must explore and determine the ways of self-regulation used by the patient and the points of their disturbances. The psychologist should subsequently describe these to the patient to make them conscious (Zeigarnik, 1986, p. 105). This is important because,

> when taking conscious measures of protection, which is a particular type of mediation of activity, there is a restoration of forms of human life activity that are adequate to reality. The need for sublimation, substituting actions, disappears. A person's actions begin to be determined by real motives, actions become purposeful, and disturbed communication is restored in forms adequate to the goals of communication. In other words, in this case, mediation turns out to be that stable personal property that begins to determine the way of life ('style') of a person, his self-esteem and vision of the world.... When activity is regulated through psychological defence mechanisms that acted on an unconscious level and ultimately made it difficult to adequately assess the situation and led to a distorted interpretation of what happened.
> 
> (Zeigarnik, 1986, p. 107)

While Zeigarnik is interested in the study and possibility of improvement of self-regulation in pathological states, there is evidence to suggest that Luria is interested in the *origin* of self-regulation and its physiological mechanisms, as well as the role of language in it. Even in brain lesions that caused an aphasia, the regulating role of speech was preserved, argues Luria. Reading Freud in parallel with Luria reveals a lot of similarities in their thinking, and each theory complements the other.

For Luria, the role of speech in regulating the activity of the child comes from the very first interactions with the parent, who dictates to the child certain 'commands'. Of course, it takes time for speech to establish the complex system of regulation, but when it is done, the power of it can dominate over 'vital instincts' (Luria, 1959, p. 71) and serve as the foundation of the regulatory role of speech in child (and, further, adult) activity. The function of speech here departs from just hearing and reproducing words.

Further investigation of this question can be evidenced in the direction Luria takes in *Speech and The Development of Mental Processes of the Child* [*Rech' i Razvitie Psikhicheskikh Protsessov u Rebenka*] (1956 in USSR, 1959 translated, 1971 Penguin book edition[47]). This is a study based on the observation of twins with learning disabilities that included slower language acquisition.

The under-developed language acquisition was not because of brain damage or organic lesions, but the child's situation had not evoked the urge for speech and communication (Luria, 1971, p. 36). In a case study, five-year-old twins[48] were placed in a situation that stimulated rapid speech development and Luria investigated how this affected the structure of mental processes. In observations, it was noticeable that the words the twins used most often were words without a constant meaning and only comprehensible in a particular situation, e.g., 'not', 'no', 'here', 'now', 'so'. Luria concluded, "as a rule our twins' speech acquired meaning only in a concrete- active situation" (Luria, 1971, p. 47). Hence the unit of their speech was not an independent word, but a word that got its meaning in the situation. Also, they used expressive exclamations, that only made sense inside the situation. Their speech was ungrammatical, with incomplete sentences without a structure.

Luria states, that normally "the child's speech begins to participate by regulating motions and actions, then secures the transition to complex forms of meaningful play and ends by becoming the most important factor in the development of conscious behaviour" (Luria, 1971, p. 52). The speech of the twins being studied "had not yet developed into an independent system and so naturally, could not fulfil the role of regulation, of planning future behaviour" (p. 52). The observation also showed that the twins understood speech that was directly related to an action or object which preoccupied them, but they did not understand speech that was not directly connected with a concrete situation and was presented in a developed narrative form. "Thus speech was completely comprehensible if it did not go beyond the bounds of the visual situation and did not become a complex stimulus which sometimes necessitated an intermediate action" (p. 56). Their independent speech and their perception of the extraneous speech was connected to the concrete actual situation. Possible reasons for this situation for Luria was "a predisposition to retardation of speech connected with phonetical impairment" and the 'twin situation' – meaning that the absence of the necessity for the development of speech as they spent most of their time together and communicated in their own idiosyncratic way.

Their play activity mirrored their language, as it was attached to concrete situations and reproduced stereotyped actions. Their play lacked an imaginative dimension and fantasy (p. 77). They could acquire the conditional meaning of objects in the concrete game, but they could not get it if it was given to them verbally (p. 79). Verbally formulated tasks for the constructive activity was also incomprehensible for the twins.

The twins were separated and one of them received a special speech training, with the aim of developing a better differentiation of sounds, better pronunciation and the acquisition of a developed speech system (p. 58). After the separation they improved their speech and their play. The children's attitude to objects began to be seen, not only when they directly engaged with them, but also in the form of projects formulated through speech (p. 91). The twin who received the speech training, however, showed slightly different results: he was able to develop what Luria called a 'theoretical attitude' towards speech (p. 103). That means the child was able to differentiate between himself and a world of objects represented by words and the structure of the language.

In other research published under the title *The Role of Speech in the Regulation of Normal and Abnormal Behavior* [*Rol' Rechi v Reguliatsii Normal'nogo i Anormal'nogo Povedeniia*] (1961), the collection of lectures that Luria gave at the University of London in 1957, he argues that the role of speech in the formation of mental processes is crucial. He is interested in finding how exactly speech can provide a regulative function.

His main postulate is that a child's mental activities are conditioned from the very beginning by social relationships with adults (Luria, 1961, p. 16). From a mother, the child acquires new modes of behaviour and new ways of organising his mental activities. This happens through the language that the mother introduces to the child. When the mother names objects for the child, she retains traces of her verbal instructions in her memory and then learns to formulate her own wishes and intentions in the inner speech. When the mother gestures towards an object and names it, the child not only acquires the designating link between the word and the object, but also acquires a position towards objects and soon begins to actively name them. In other words, a child occupies the position of the mother (identifies with her) and soon the words she uses play a part in regulating his own activities, "by using speech for himself, he alters the relative strength of the stimuli acting upon him and adapts his behavior to the influences thus modified" (p. 20).

The study showed that when facing difficulties, children of three or four years old seek an adult who can explain to them how to get over the difficulty they have, and will not act before the adult steps in. Children of five to seven, on the other hand, attempt to solve difficulties if no help is given, and this evokes "an outburst of active speech, addressed in part to the adult present but chiefly to anyone" (p. 33). This outburst of speech, Luria noticed, performs a practical function helping a child to find ways out of difficult situations. He calls it 'verbal orientation to surroundings'. Sometime later, at the age of seven, these speech outbursts disappear, but they are not gone, as they locate 'inside' forming what is called internal speech, "an invariable part of the thought-process" (p. 34). Luria concludes, that to evaluate the development of the child is not to give him or her tasks and see results, but to see how much a child can make use of the help of an adult and apply it to their independent activity thereafter (p. 41).

Through the series of experiments Luria and colleagues tried to find out how and when speech begins to regulate the activity of the child. The conclusion he came to is that

> *the regulatory function is steadily transferred from the impulse side of the speech to the analytic system of elective significative connections which are produced by speech.* Moreover, and this is most interesting, it simultaneously shifts *from the external to the internal speech of the child.*
>
> (p. 92, Luria's emphases)

In the light of this work, we can say that the slower development of the speech and play in the twin couple happened also because they missed having a supporting adult. In the foreword, Luria indicated that the twins were the youngest members in a large family with much older siblings. The parents did not devote much time to doing activities with them and they were predominantly spending most of their time on their own. One more thing that also attracted my attention was the fact that the speech of their mother still suffered from remnants of "complex phonetical impairment" (Luria, 1971, p. 39). Therefore, the way she verbalized objects for the twins was phonematically distorted.

We can trace back the idea of the importance of the phonematic component in the organisation of the psyche to Freud's work *On Aphasia* (1891). Freud suggests that there are two elements of perceptions of words: visual and auditory, which organize the work of the mental apparatus. He also highlights that perception is inseparable from the process of association, and they both operate together (p. 57). In the scheme below:

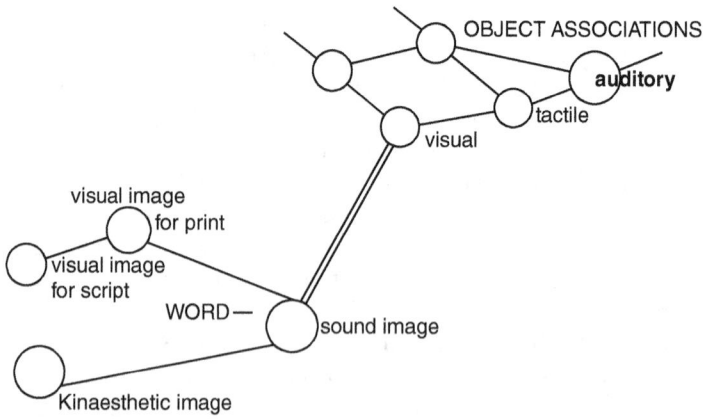

*Figure 4.1* Psychological schema of the word concept (Freud, 1891)

The word concept appears as a closed complex of images, the object concept as an open one. The word concept is linked to the concept of the object via the sound image only. Among the object associations, the visual ones play a part similar to that played by the sound image among the word associations. The connections of the word sound image with object associations other than the visual are not presented in this schema (Freud, 1891, p. 77)

The distinction between the image and sound components of words is important and will continue to organize Freud's thinking in his work on jokes and subsequently on the unconscious, where he will use other terms, word-presentation and thing-presentation,[49] to explain different ways of how perception of objects is stored in our mind. These terms will be used consistently in his later works to explain the functioning of the mind, both in the 'topographical model' and the 'structural model'.

Another work where this is brought forth is the *Interpretation of Dreams* (1900), where he argues that in dream work some of the presentations are leftovers of the acoustic presentations – 'auditory images' (Freud, 1900, p. 49). This idea also appears in *The Ego and the Id* (1923), where Freud presents the scheme of the id-ego-super ego, where the ego wears 'a cap of hearing' (p. 24) – the 'auditory' component of the ego. However, it is not about what the ego hears, but about auditory leftovers of words that populate the unconscious and become a part of the mind. In the same work Freud also connects the origin of the super ego in what we hear from our parents:

> [I]t is as impossible for the super-ego as for the ego to disclaim its origin from things heard: for it is a part of the ego and remains accessible to consciousness by way of these word-presentations (concepts, abstractions).
> (Freud, 1923, p. 51)

Overall, the unconscious is populated by the residues of what we heard and by acoustic presentations of objects that were provided to us by their signifiers. "The visual components of word-presentations are secondary, acquired through reading, and may begin to be left on one side.... In essence a word is after all the mnemic residue of a word that has been heard" (Freud, 1923, p. 20).

For the twins in Luria's study, this process of 'population of the mind' was stifled, because of the lack of adult participation in it and because of the phonemic lack. That directly impacted upon their mental activity, which directly affected the way they played and constructed their actions. Being surrounded by adults in the kindergarten on a regular basis improved their speech. That restored their capacity for self-regulation.

It is clear, from his research interests, that Luria was indeed interested in the formation of mental apparatus, both in consciousness and the way it is regulated by language and mental processes like attention and thinking. In Freudian terms, Luria is concerned with the psychic (mental) apparatus and metapsychology. In the first chapter of his book *Language and Cognition* (1981) he places language as of "decisive importance for the further development of human conscious activity" (Luria, 1981, p. 27). Therefore, to study complex thinking and other mental processes is impossible for Luria without considering the role of language. However, what is missing in Luria's vocabulary in this book is the notion of the ego or the self, an individual constellation of the sense of "I". Instead, he places a capacity for self- regulation via language at the place where the ego should be. Self-regulation for Luria in its function serves the function of the ego and super-ego in Freudian terms.

It is quite understandable that after many years of persecution for his relations with psychoanalysis, Luria would not be eager to include such terminology in his writing. At the same time, for Luria, as well as for Zeigarnik, the notion of ego is not as important as that of the idea of consciousness, and in the strict sense they never went beyond Freud's first topographical model of the mind. Therapeutic encounter, as we've seen, for Luria is in the process of the development of the language and social expansion of the twins. Can we combine Luria's ideas with Freud's to make them useful for the psychotherapeutic encounter? To me, it expands for us Freud's formula "Where id was there ego shall be" (Freud, 1933, p. 80). However, I suggest, if we stay in the dimension of metapsychology, rather than ego-psychology, the role of language in self-regulation as suggested by Luria, will nuance this formula with an extra meaning.

The first and foremost function of the ego is to connect with reality. Through multiple encounters with the world, it attempts to release the tension of the drive and set out relationships with objects. The child then begins to obtain language – serving as mediator between body and reality. Words as language units 'populate' the mind and serve as a residual of objects in the memory and presentations for drives. Processes of storage and expression, thus, simultaneously occur in the 'psychic apparatus' and organize the flow of thinking. At first libidinal drives, id, prevail due to the inefficiency of the mediation available to a child, and games like 'fort-da', rituals and repetitions serve as regulating mechanisms. Of course, the parent plays a big part in regulation and navigation of the child's drives. With the help of a parent, through words and expansion of the symbolic universe of language, a child sets up certain descriptions of the drives and attributes them to himself/herself. The ego here, being a symbolic mediator itself, creates repetitions that becomes 'characteristics' of the child. This acquisition of the ego is linked to language, and language begins to regulate activity through the repetition of the patterns of the ego. At first it is a regulatory mechanism, and only later identification with regulatory processes sets up the space for a child to become an I, addressed by the adult as someone being 'lovely', 'like a grandfather' etc. However, argues Freud, the ego in neurosis or psychosis does not handle the negotiation with reality,

[i]n both cases it serves the desire for power of the id, which will not allow itself to be dictated to by reality ... in neurosis a piece of reality is avoided by a sort of flight, whereas in psychosis it is remodelled.

(1924, p. 185)

For neurotics, the identifications of the ego begin to dominate over the mediation function of the ego between drives and reality. The ego loses 'healthy' self-regulation in the attempt to negotiate between id and reality and instead of a search for various mediators it creates symptoms (Freud, 1923, p. 55). A similar process is happening when the mind deals with psychotic breakdown – mediators (words) become overcharged with libidinal energy in order to compensate for the ego, which falls apart under the pressures of the id or super-ego (Freud, 1924a, p. 183).

Through the lens of the notion of regulation via language as suggested by Luria, the 'talking cure' in both psychosis and neurosis appears to be not only helpful via insights and revisiting the past. Talking as a process itself has a curative potential through the intimate link between the function of the ego and the language. The development of the language of the patient, faced with the need to communicate with the therapist, may in fact, play a greater role in the therapy, than insights or interpretations. This sheds light on why Zeigarnik saw the therapeutic potential of the pathopsychology procedure, and the overall therapeutic encounter, based on the self- regulation idea. Also, I see Luria's formulations on the role of language in the regulation of activity as a productive elaboration of Freud's ideas, the vicissitudes of psychoanalysis that had to negotiate with the reality of the Soviet censorship and Stalinist model of science.

\*

Overall, considering the archival research discussed earlier in the chapter, we can place the shift to neuropsychology and the 'abandonment' of psychoanalysis by Luria in the plane of the personal, rather than theoretical choice. The inclusion of a persecutor in Luria's case, introducing for almost 15 years doubt over the scientific validity and purity of his work, created a traumatic dimension in the relationship between Luria and psychoanalytic theory. The trauma was, nevertheless, not linked to Freud's ideas, but to the discordance of authorities with Freud.

Through the study of his scientific interests, it is also apparent that, in the strict sense, the shift to neuropsychology never happened fully, and Luria continued to practice an interdisciplinary approach to the mind with an emphasis on the psychology, rather than physiology, of it. Also, through his experiments, psychoanalytic theory was elaborated and at the same time continued to preserve Freud's early interests in studying aphasia and his later interests in the role of the ego in mental functioning.

## Notes

1. The impact of psychoanalysis on the further development of the theoretical and clinical views of Alexander Luria is recognized as well by Russian historian Bogdanchikov, however, more as a passing comment in the footnote: "It seems that without the influence of psychoanalysis, all subsequent general psychological and neuropsychological constructions of A. R. Luria would not have been so carefully thoughtful and convincing – both for A. R. Luria himself, and for all scientific communities" (2002, p. 84).
2. The predecessor of this study is Luria's experimental work with children done together with Vygotsky. Proctor (2020) gives a full account of this. Conducted between 1923 and 1936, a time of relative freedom of thought and progress in pedology, these observations and experiments focused on the future citizens of the Soviet state, and therefore with understanding the processes of child development. Luria and Vygotsky's focus was on the role of language, play and historical context for mental development.
3. GARF, f. R4737, op. 2, 1509
4. Perhaps, not surprisingly, Luria's findings were distorted by his own pupils, who shifted to the 'empty' brain-scanning procedure, where the subject (in the psychoanalytic sense) is lost, or, perhaps, has never even been present.
5. Or to be specific, GARF files now stored in Yalutorovsk, a town in Tyumen oblast, 2,000km from Moscow. If not for COVID that opened minds to the digitalisation of documents, and the kindness of archivists who work there, I would never have been able to access these folders.
6. GARF, f.P-9506, o.15, d.81a, p. 105.
7. GARF, f.P-9506, o.15, d.81a, p. 118.
8. GARF, f.P-9506, o.15, d.81a, p. 59.
9. GARF, f.P-9506, o.15, d.81a, p. 103.
10. GARF, f.P-9506, o.15, d.81a, p. 103.
11. GARF, f.P-9506, o.15, d.81a, p. 60.
12. Victor Kolbanovskii, a psychologist who in 1936 wrote a critical article about 'psychotechnics' from the Marxist standpoint, that led to its liquidation. After he graduated from the Institute of the Red Professors, he become a head of the Institute of Psychology 1932–1937 and most likely served as a link between the party and the institute. A short memoire about him is in Platonov, K. K., *Moi lichnyye vstrechi na velikoy doroge zhizni (Vospominaniya starogo psikhologa)*, M.: Institut psikhologii RAN, 2005, p. 194–204.
13. I could not find anyone with this surname in academic circles of that time, which is most likely the sign that Shimbelev was a 'red' professor.
14. From the text of the commission Plotnikov appears as a party representative.
15. There are two ways in which Smirnov is mentioned, one is comrade, and one is professor. The initials of comrade Smirnov were M. T. but I did not find information about anyone with these initials. At that time Kolbanovskii worked with Anatolii Smirnov, psychologist, statesman and politician, former specialist in pedology, who had to denounce his views as everyone else in 1936. At the time of the commission, he was a professor in the Moscow Pedagogical Institute. An article about his path is in the MSU Faculty of Psychology, http://psy.msu.ru/people/smirnov_aa.html Perhaps, when it is Prof. Smirnov, it is Anatolii, while comrade Smirnov is someone called M. T.
16. This is the first time this letter is referenced in the research dedicated to Luria. Translation from Russian into English is mine.
17. Here, and further in the text of the letter, the emphases are mine.

18 Tubetzkoy was a linguist and historian whose teachings formed a nucleus of the Prague School of Structural Linguistics. In the years 1922–1938 he lived in Vienna. He was a friend and colleague of Roman Jakobson, and a follower of Ferdinand de Saussure. The work Luria supposedly presented was published in the book *Grundzuege der Phonologie* (1939) (*Principles of Phonology*. The English translation of this book is here: https://monoskop.org/images/7/73/Trubetzkoy_NS_Principles_of_Phonology.pdf). Ideas on the phonematic structure of the language became an important part of Luria's work. He refers to Trubetzkoy in his work on aphasia, language and consciousness.

We can trace the idea of the impact of the language, and especially its phonetic component on the functioning of the mind in Luria's work on the formation of children's mind (his speech at the congress in London in 1965) and his work on aphasia.

19 GARF, f.P-9506, o.15, d.81a, pp. 113–117.
20 GARF, f.P-9506, o.15, d.81a, pp. 78–79.
21 GARF, f.P-9506, o.15, d.81a, pp. 60–65.
22 A discussion of Luria's expedition and its outcomes see in Proctor (2020), chapter 'The Primitive' and Yasnitsky and van der Veer (2015), chapter 'Did Uzbeks have illusion? The Luria-Koffka controversy of 1932'.
23 GARF, f.P-9506, o.15, d.81a, pp. 66–67.
24 GARF, f.P-9506, o.15, d.81a, pp. 67–68.
25 However the 'substantial corrections' in Luria's work were related to the ongoing suspicion towards him as a scientist and multiple references to Freud and Jung in this work.
26 GARF, f.P-9506, o.15, d. 81a, pp. 70–71.
27 GARF, f.P-9506, o.15, d.81a, p. 44.
28 Supposedly a secretary.
29 Sergei Kaftanov was at that time Chairman of the VAK.
30 Apparently Alexei Gagarin, a philosopher, was a vice chairman of the Higher Attestation Comission (VAK). Like Kolbanovskii, he graduated from the Institute of Red Professors and for many years was a dean of the Philosophy Faculty in MSU. More about his career path is at https://philos.msu.ru/node/1338
31 It is interesting to note, that I have heard the same argument from academic psychologists of the 'Russian' tradition. Mistakes of youth – a common expression, serves here as a template for the logical error and as a result of uncritical thinking. On the other occasion, when speaking about someone talented or even genius, it is emphasized that he or she was interested in the topic from their young age – serving as a solid support for the genuineness of their interest.
32 GARF, f.P-9506, o.15, d.81a, p.45
33 The presenter refers here to the fact that Luria has conducted experiments in physiology without physiological education. For us it again argues for the nature of Luria's interest, which was never primarily physiological, even at times when he measured physiological reactions.
34 Although it might be a mere speculation, it looks like Tbilisi Institute was under 'protection' supposedly because Stalin was from Georgia. Or members of commission were afraid to made 'mistakes' themselves by not acknowledging the hight level of expertise of Georgian psychologists.
35 GARF, f.P-9506, o.15, d.81a, p.47
36 GARF, f.P-9506, o.15, d.81a, p. 53.

37 In the stenograph of the commission held on 8 June 1939 comrade Plotnikov a mention that Luria's current dissertation contain 'methodological mistakes' of a 'Freudian kind' (GARF, f.P-9506, ë.15, d.81a, p. 92).
38 GARF, f.P-9506, o.15, d.81a, p. 51.
39 GARF, f.P-9506, o.15, d.81a, p. 53.
40 GARF, f.P-9506, o.15, d.81a, p. 55.
41 GARF, f.P-9506, o.15, d.81a, p. 118.
42 GARF, f.P-9506, o.15, d.81a, p. 38.
43 GARF, f.P-9506, o.15, d.81a, p. 9.
44 GARF, f.P-9506, o.15, d.81a, p. 3.
45 GARF, f.P-9506, o.15, d.81a, p. 2.
46 The idea of mediation, or symbolic mediation, developed by Vygotsky means that mental processes are always mediated by symbols, serving as tools for the mind. Vygotsky stated the social origin of consciousness and emphasized the determination of consciousness by speech and regulation of it by the sign. The word is a basic tool for mediation and thus for Vygotsky is an intermediary for self- regulation. An example of the symbolic mediation in Freud's work is the Fort-Da game, where sounds play the role of an object (mother). (The summary is given on the basis of the article Ulybina, E. V. (2004) Sign mediation in cultural-historical theory and psychoanalysis. *Psychological Journal, 25(6)*: 64–73)
47 The editor of the book in the Introduction suggests the reader skips the first chapter (methodology) and starts with the second instead, and only after reading the whole book to return to the first chapter. "All that - and I must leave it at that – is the background against which I see Professor Luria's experiment in this book. What I must not do is suggest that it is the background against which the author himself sees it; this he has set out rigorously and fully in his first chapter. (But it is a difficult statement for readers not acquainted with the kind of psychological theories he discusses: I recommend for such readers that they begin reading at chapter 2, taking on trust that first paragraph on page 34, and returning to read chapter 1 when they have read the rest of the book)" (Luria, 1971, p. 13).
48 The twins did not speak till they were two years old and then only learned "mama" and "papa". At four years they only used undifferentiated sounds in play and communication (p. 39). By the age of five they had learned a range of simple words and their speech was phonematically impaired.
49 A bridge between Freud's studies on aphasia and the unconscious see in Strachey's Appendix C: Words and Things to *The Unconscious* (1915).

Chapter 5

# The Soviet unconscious
## Uznadze, Bassin and others

In this chapter I return to the histories of Dmitry Uznadze and Filipp Bassin, two leading voices in Soviet studies on the unconscious. Although they deserve a book each, especially given they both remain understudied in Russian-speaking and English academia, this chapter will look only at specific moments in their careers when they engaged with the notion of the unconscious and the culmination of their effort – The International Symposium on the Unconscious, an event held in Tbilisi in 1979 and the four volumes of the symposium papers.

Through reading the main monographs of Bassin and Uznadze, I aim to show how, the notion of the 'Soviet unconscious' based on Uznadze's theory of set and established by Bassin as an alternative to Freud was not that much different from Freud. The criticism of Freud that appeared in their work is due to political reasons, and should be read not as a critique, but as a disguise technique that was used by Bassin to keep the discussion about psychoanalysis alive after 1956.

This brings us back to the question of the vicissitudes of psychoanalysis, and specifically to the notion of the unconscious, that despite changes brought by the Soviet era, the shift to an experimental approach and the need to be negated or disguised under the critique, preserved its meaning throughout the period in question. I am curious about the Soviet contribution to the theory of psychoanalysis. Can we learn something from reading Uznadze and Bassin today?

Materials for this chapter are taken predominantly from the archival documents I obtained from GARF, mentions of Uznadze and Bassin in the Soviet press (years 1920–1980, accessed via the *EastView* database) and in academic journals *Voprosy Psikhologii* and *Voprosy Filosofii* (years 1950–1980, issues obtained in the Senate House library and in the UCL SSEES library). It also engages with their main monographs, as well as details about their work from the secondary literature. For some biographical details and the discussion of their input into Soviet psychology see Imedadze (2009), Ketchuashvili (2014), Kozulin (1989), Ladaria (2014), Yasnitsky (2009, 2019).

## 'The struggle' with Uznadze and the theory of set

"Psychology appears to us as the science of the concrete mental life of the subject, and not as the science of the abstract mental phenomena" (Uznadze, 1966, p. 200).

It was reiterated multiple times by Bassin (1968) that Uznadze's theory of set is a Soviet alternative to Freud and lies at the core of the Soviet theory of the unconscious. In this part of the chapter, I am reading through the main monograph of Uznadze, dedicated to the study of set, to explore its relationship to the Freudian notion of the unconscious.

Through the observation and interpretation of parapraxes, mistakes, dreams and free associations, Freud formulated several special characteristics of the unconscious (1901, 1915). Unlike the conscious mind, it does not operate according to laws of time and space and, as well as rational knowledge about laws of reality, does not recognize negation; there is no such thing as ambivalence there, no doubt, no degrees of certainty (Freud, 1915, p. 185). The nucleus of the unconscious consists of the representations of drives, or wishful impulses (p. 185). Overall, the unconscious knows little about external reality and can only become cognizable when dreaming or through neurosis. Discharge from the unconscious 'passes into the somatic' (p. 186). Nevertheless, unconscious activity has a huge impact on our being. Our ego is formed to be partially unconscious, as well as our super ego. That brings a completely new dynamic for our mental functioning, from everyday life activity and choices to the formation of 'unwanted' phenomena, like excessive emotional reactions or symptoms. Hence, we always observe 'leftovers' or 'effects' of the unconscious, conclude Freud, and we cannot study it directly.

The set, on the other hand, as presented in the Soviet literature, was studied experimentally. In fact, it was deduced from a series of phenomena, observed in experiments that explored various illusions of shape, weight, sound, light, etc. This is an interesting detail to note – that the theory of set is constructed theoretically as a hypothesis that could explain various illusions observed experimentally. One may get an illusion that the set itself was studied experimentally, an important illusion to keep alive, especially when Pavlov's experiments with dogs dominated the field. For that experimental shield, it is difficult not to overestimate the meaning that theory of set had for the discussion around the unconscious in 1950–1980.

Dmitry Uznadze (1886–1950) was called 'father' of a Georgian school of psychology and a person who brought

> a new understanding of how action is rooted in the personality and of how behaviour is regulated, the discovery of their psychological dimension and the establishment of an original method for research into unconscious forms of mental activity [that] marked the beginning of a new and remarkably promising stage on the road to a knowledge of mental processes.
>
> (Ketchuashvili, 2014, p. 1)

Uznadze lived and worked in Tbilisi, Georgia (later Georgian SSR). He studied philosophy at Leipzig University (1909), history and philology in Kharkhiv (1913) and then returned to Tbilisi (1918) where he founded the department of psychology. The Georgian school of psychology was relatively independent from the capital, partly because it was held in Georgian, a language that was unavailable for the authorities, and partly because of the distance – it was too far away to be under constant oversight.

Uznadze had a wide range of interests – he studied "the psychology of thought and speech, perception, attention and the will, and works in the field of differential genetic psychology, the psychology of labour and the psychology of art" (Ketchuashvili, 2014, p. 9). His work was concerned also with developmental psychology and the role of language in thinking processes; he was interested in the phenomena of dreams, studied representations and perception.[1] A lot of his work, however, was published in Georgian first, hence remained inaccessible for the Russian reader up until the 1960s.

The book fully dedicated to the theory of set was actually published in Russian only in 1961 and "it can hardly be considered accessible to Russian readers who are interested in the theory of set" (Imedadze, 2009, p. 7) as only 1,000 copies were printed. Its original year of publication in Georgian was 1949, therefore it would not be surprising that many public readers discovered Uznadze for the first time from the newspaper. Enthusiasts of public criticism did not pass by Uznadze's set theory. In 1952 *Literaturnaia gazeta* (March, No. 30) published a critical article by D. Gedevanishvili, denouncing Uznadze and his theory of set for being idealistic, following Freud and rejecting Pavlov. In 1956 *Voprosy psikhologii* published another attack by A. A. Kuteliia, where he criticized Dmitry Uznadze and his theory of set for their idealistic nature and interest in the unconscious (Kuteliia, 1956). The attack was not personal, as Uznadze was dead by that time, and perhaps signify that his ideas were seen as influential, hence posed a threat to the Pavlovization campaign.

For academics, of course, it was different. Articles about the set appeared in *Voprosy Psikhologii* before the official book translation. Similarly, in Bassin's articles we find references to Uznadze's work from the mid-1950s, and even as early as 1945 we find a mention of the manuscript dedicated to the 'Role of the Psychological Notion of the Set for Neurophysiology'.[2] While we know already that Luria chose to defend his work in Tbilisi University in 1938, and remained lifelong friends with Uznadze, he does not discuss the theory of set in his writings to any depth. In Zeigarnik's writings, the theory of set is mentioned on several occasions, but merely in the outline of various studies of the mind. The circulation of Uznadze's ideas in Moscow and Leningrad, perhaps, depended also on the scientific agenda of those times.

It will be informative to let Uznadze's critics provide us with insights on the wrongdoings of the theory of set. Kuteliia exposes the substitution that Uznadze made in his writings, when "he changed notions such as 'subconscious' and 'unconscious' with other terms, ... and after all calls it 'psychology of set'" (Kuteliia, 1956, p. 37). Indeed, in the 1920s and 1930s it was still called "theory of the unconscious psychological set". Other critics find that the set conflicts with reflex theory and reflexology (Mdivani, Kechuashvili and Nadirashvili, 1956, p. 144–152); as we will see from reading Uznadze's monograph, this is in fact an accurate observation, primarily because he stood for the impossibility of generalization of observations from experimental studies of animal behaviour to humans. Even though Uznadze did not necessarily point towards Pavlov's dogs when rejecting the value of such studies, it was enough for his critics to 'build a case' against him. Another point of discontent is that he considered the set to be a more complex structure than a reflex. Gedevanishvili adds to this, that Uznadze does not recognize the direct reflection of external reality on the mind, but sees it as mediated by the set. Also, the significant role of Freud and absence of mention of Pavlov in Uznadze's monograph makes it clear that Uznadze is an "idealistic, bourgeois" psychologist (Gedevanishvili, 1952).

To be able to bring Uznadze to the wider audience after 1950, one of his colleagues Prangishvili[3] had to adopt the same strategy as Bassin when discussing Uznadze's studies on the unconscious. It took him years for to restore the reputation of Uznadze and to negotiate his 'separateness' from Freud. This was managed in a similar way as in 1958 in the Freud Session, where it was decided to open a new chapter of Soviet research into the unconscious, different from the idealist Freud. A discussion around the theory of set in further issues of *Voprosy Psikhologii* throughout the years 1956 (n5, n6); 1958 (n4); 1966 (n1); 1967 (n1) resulted in some kind of agreement in 1967 (n4) that Uznadze was, after all, a Soviet psychologist. Meanwhile, in 1966, his book *The Psychology of Set* was translated into English and prepared for publication in New York. Published in The International Behavioural Sciences series, this book, alongside with Zeigarnik's *Abnormal Psychology*, was put on library shelves that very likely were never reached by readers interested in psychoanalysis.

Researchers into Uznadze claim the methodological uniqueness of his view. For him,

> external and internal factors do not directly cause behaviour and, consequently, the related psychic processes, but indirectly – through the set; first a set arises as a modification, an adjustment of the holistic subject manifested in the readiness of his psychophysical functions to perform a certain activity, after which concrete behavior based on it is carried out.
> (Imedadze, 2009, p. 8)

For Uznadze, there can be no direct impact of external onto internal reality, differentiating his view from that "blind adherence to the postulate of directness" that was shared by all classical psychology as well as new theoretical movements such as Gestalt psychology and behaviourism. He based his views on the 'mediate nature of the psyche' (Imedadze, 2009, p. 8). Uznadze's view of the mind was of the holistic kind (Imedadze, 2009; Ketchuashvili, 2014) and his interest was to see activity as a result of the interaction of visceral, motor and psychic reactions, where the set – a dynamic construction – played an important role in shaping this activity. Perhaps, his holistic approach to the unconscious was the most developed amongst Soviet psychologists and physiologists. One may say that the dream of Freud that some physiological ground will be found for the unconscious in further generations of scientists was realized in these Soviet studies.

The difference between the Freudian unconscious and Uznadze's set is

> seriously discussed in many studies (F.B. Bassin, I.T. Bzhalava, V.L. Kakabadze, A.E. Sheroziia, and others). There is especially rich material on this subject in the well-known fundamental four-volume set of materials from the international conference on the unconscious held in Tbilisi (1979).
>
> (Imedadze, 2009, p. 26)

They are normally focused on two moments. The first distinctive feature of the set is that it is not just the negative of the conscious. The second is that unlike the 'id', the set operates according to the reality principle, and not the pleasure principle. In that sense, the theory of set is much closer to the dynamic unconscious than it might look at the first sight, with the emphasis on the role of drives. Even the notion of unconscious phantasy as formulated by Melanie Klein includes all characteristics of the set and especially that 'mediate nature of psyche' highlighted as a unique position of Uznadze.

I suggest seeing the theory of set as a productive elaboration of the concept of the unconscious, in a way specific to Soviet psychology. That includes the attempt to experimentally capture the unconscious and study its role in the formation of the character/personality and the action/activity. Close reading and discussion of *The Psychology of Set* (1966) will support the above suggestion.

The definition of 'set' is not straightforward. The set is "some form of internal state, which prepares a person for perception" (Uznadze, 1966, p. 8). I think the English word 'set' does not fully translate the Russian word '*ustanovka*', which I would explain via a combination of meanings held by the words 'settings', as we understand the settings of a device to be configured in a special way, and 'attitude', indicating the predisposition for perception. Importantly, the set does not relate to the phenomena of consciousness (p. 10), but overall influences the activity of the individual.

In the introduction Uznadze explains what the unconscious is:

1   It is constituted by repression.

> Let us assume that a subject develops some desire that he regards as unsuitable, or perhaps even shameful, for some reason or other. What

happens in such a case? The psychology of the unconscious here falls back upon the concept of repression, and it is assumed that the subject 'represses' the desire from his consciousness, not eradicating it once and for all, but merely relegating it to the depths of his unconscious. In this repressed, and not unconscious, state, the desire is not consciously previewed or experienced by the subject, but it is not forever disposed of. And so, according to the theory, this is how one very considerable part of the unconscious mind is created.

(Uznadze, 1966, ix)

2   It overdetermines the work of the mind.

Being an integral state, the set lies at the basis of the absolutely determinate mental phenomena arising in consciousness. It does not in any way follow these phenomena, but, on the contrary, it may be said to prepare for their appearance, to determine their course and composition.

(p. 10)

Apparently so far this is not different from the psychoanalytic view of the unconscious.

Very soon after, Uznadze expresses his view that the main problem of psychology lies in the absence of the mediator between external reality and internal reality:

It seems to me that modern bourgeois psychology is entirely based on a dogmatically perceived postulate, not previously verified and not susceptible to criticism, according to which objective reality spontaneously and immediately influences the conscious mind and, by this spontaneous link, determines its activity.

(p. 18)

Also, for Uznadze the source of activity is different, as it comes from the 'inside', rather being determined by external reality. He proposes two fundamental conditions of activity: the need and the situation (pp. 24, 26). Needs are divided into substantive and functional. He is critical of the consideration of the behaviour of the higher monkeys in anthropomorphic terms (p. 25) and highlights the abstract intellectual needs as a specific group of needs arising in humans. Intellectual needs are considered as further complications of substantive needs.

The formation of the set happens when the internal meets the external, "for a set to develop, it is essential that a corresponding [to the need] situation be present, in which it assumes a definite, concrete character" (p. 27). This happens with the active role of repetition (p. 40). So we can say that the set is a repetition of the situation of the realization of the need. These statements correspond to Freud's idea on the vicissitudes of the drives. Being fully unconscious, drives emerge in the body from the pulsation of the life of our organs and create the tension that appears on the surface of our mind (psyche), yet without an object. The object for the drive is found through the realization of that tension, and 'offered' at first by external reality. If there is no enabling environment for the drive to be realized, it is postponed or redirected to another object (Freud, 1915). To keep the object close that has given us the release of the drive's tension, we develop something called 'love', argues Freud. In this case, love repeatedly captures the drive and the object together. Through the repetition of certain actions from a very young age, we achieve the realization of the drives. The mystery of mind for psychoanalysis is precisely in the moment of choice: how do certain objects become more favourable than others, why do we keep attaching ourselves to certain kinds of objects? This question becomes even more important when we exit the consulting room and go to the shopping centre, where certain objects seem to be already charged with our desire (Salecl, 2011). The unconscious continues to live its life of favours and choices without our conscious participation in it. For Uznadze this is what represents the set – the unconscious part of the structure, directing our actions without our conscious knowledge, and at the same time being a mediator between external and internal reality.

Let's continue our reading of Uznadze's monograph. An interesting phenomenon of the set occurred in more than half of the cases. Once the set was established in one sensory region, say visual field, irradiation[4] of it to haptic and muscular spheres was observed, and he found the same phenomena occurring in all sensory regions (Uznadze, 1966, pp. 32–34).[5] In other words, the set was spread through invisible channels taking over perceptions without control of the individual. Based on that he formulated his 'disagreement' with Freud's statement that unconscious and conscious processes are fundamentally identical. Perhaps this is an example of the same disguise technique followed by criticism leading to the same conclusions as the criticized author:

> I think if we could establish that the mental content of the unconscious is not that usually associated with conscious life but still not radically separated from it, we would possess a weapon which would enable us to obtain a much deeper understanding of the true state of affairs.
>
> (p. 39)

In fact, for Freud the unconscious was never just non-conscious and from the beginning (1900) he insisted on the radical difference of these two dimensions of the mind and formulated their difference (1915).

The establishment of the set was not identical for every participant. A group of individuals who always give a correct estimate of the size of the experimental objects is of interest to us. In this case, assumes Uznadze, we are dealing with persons lacking the internal directing power and being extremely extravert (p. 49). That might indicate that such persons are clear from pre-set expectations and able to correct their experiences according to the changing environment. By contrast, another group of individuals developed a persistent set leading to the return of the illusion. Their initial response after the critical exposures was correction of set and they gave right answers. However, after some time they returned to the initial set (p. 55). These responses show the extent to which the reality of the external world can influence established set. In a way, the same question was at the core of Freud's attempt to diagnose between neuroses and psychoses in their relation to reality (Freud, 1924a) pointing that the correction of the individual structure by demands of external reality is limited; it is only to a certain extent, and only with a temporary effect.

For Uznadze the set is at the core of how we see ourselves, defining how and when we are going to act.

> We may accordingly conclude that each one of us carries within himself an innumerable multitude of sets fixed in the course of life which, when activated by a suitable condition, regulate the working of our mind in the corresponding direction.
>
> (Uznadze, 1966, p. 60)

The dynamic nature of the mind, responding in a certain way to specific circumstances, is closely linked to speech. For Uznadze, verbal symbols, as he puts it, "while possessing no true meaning of their own, represent to us certain forms of stimulation" (p. 109), and therefore organize verbal reality. In other words, sets can be activated and transformed via speech.

"The development of conscious mental processes is preceded by a state which cannot in any degree be regarded as a nonmental, purely physiological state" (p. 90). This idea corresponds to the psychoanalytic view of the relations between the conscious and the unconscious. It is not only in parapraxes and jokes that the unconscious reveals itself. Any action we observe, and this is the part that makes the process of psychoanalysis hard, can reveal the unconscious structures behind it. Even if the action appears rational or coincidental, it contains the element of unconscious determination. A constant process of revealing the truth about one's own reasons, understanding the drives behind own actions outside of the consulting room makes everyday life especially hard. The presupposition of the unconscious meaning behind actions that on the surface appear as conscious decisions brings us to limitations of conscious ability in regulating our own activity. This is one of the narcissistic wounds that psychoanalysis is famous for: we are not masters in our own houses.

Uznadze, in that sense, was even more Freudian than Freud, as for him every action is determined by the set, hence connected to the unconscious. This totality, on the other hand, brings us to the question to what extent Uznadze's experiments can provide psychoanalysis with insights, while the latter deals only with specific forms of the unconscious – dreams, parapraxes, symptoms? The answer to this, again, lies in the totality of the unconscious as we see it developed in Lacanian and Kleinian psychoanalysis. For Uznadze it is also important that the set is built on what he calls the 'idea', based on images/perceptions of the object and verbal representations. His experiments have shown that ideas play an important role in forming certain sets, although their strength is less than those built on 'real' objects (pp. 121–122). This is "a new stratum which can be found only in subjects working with ideas, notions, or thoughts" (p. 122).

A thought appears when the obstacle interrupts the action towards the satisfaction of "the theoretical, perceptual need" (p. 133) and is impossible without what Uznadze calls 'objectivization' – the specific act of "turning an object or phenomenon included in a chain of human activity into a special, independent object of observation" (p. 117). "In a sphere of activity where there is no objectivization, there can be no true thought"[6] (p. 133). This ability to recognize external objects as phenomena in internal reality is supported by perception. The intrinsic connection between thought and objectivation, as well as the emergence of thought in the situation of the obstacle corresponds to the views expressed by Freud in his early work (1911). Angelini (1988) in his book on *Psychoanalysis in Russia*, suggests that Uznadze's notion of 'objectification' is similar to Freud's 'secondary process' (p. 141).

As results of the study of the set were varied, a classification of 'types' of people was formulated to describe differences in responses. Uznadze named them as 'dynamic', 'static' and 'variable'. Although it appears as a typology, this classification is more of a descriptive character, and represents results obtained during the series of experiments. The main differences between those groups are 1. the constancy of the set in the 'static' group is higher as well as 2. irradiation from one sensory sphere to others. In other words, the set establishes itself more rigidly and once appeared, it irradiates and hence fixates the perception accordingly. This is like something that Freud notices about neurotic structure, which is based on 'wishful' thinking and fantasy, rather than reality, and has the power to distort perception and thinking according to the wish. This is not to co-ordinate Uznadze's typology with the diagnostic structures of psychoanalysis, but to highlight the explanatory potential of it.

Uznadze studied the set in psychopathology. His views on the nature of mental disturbances are very close to those expressed by Zeigarnik:

> It is now firmly established that the basis of psychotic and psychoneurotic state is not a definite anomaly of some special character, nor a disease of specific mental functions, but an integral process affecting the diseased personality as a whole.
>
> (Uznadze, 1966, p. 155)

The integral structure of the personality – this is what gets affected and affects the course of the mental disturbance.

The experimental study of the set in patients with schizophrenia shows that their sets are predominantly coarse, static, rigid, irradiated and stable. That is, Uznadze notices, not specific to patients with schizophrenia, as in the group of 'normal' patients he found the same results. The difference is in the process of the objectivization, which, according to Uznadze, is less available or not available at all for patients with schizophrenia (p. 170).

A finding specific to the set in patients with hysteria is their variability, depending on the condition of the patient. Also Uznadze discovered that sets based on imagined ideas develop much more easily and stronger, than in 'healthy' persons (p. 186). This is unusual, as normally sets stimulated by imagination are less strong than those provoked by real situations, and proves "the important role of the imagined ideas in the mental activity of hysterical subjects", and "these 'ideas' are not mental states differentiated psychologically from perception" (p. 187). These findings are very much in tune with Freudian ideas on hysteria, where a subject suffers from reminiscences. In Freud's view, for the hysterical subject the idea is no less important than the perceptive trace of the real event (Breuer and Freud, 1893).

Overall, the most important component of mental functioning for Uznadze turned out to be objectivization. This is the process that helps the mind to adjust to changes in reality, to correct sets and to navigate activity through recognition of the objects of the outside world and separating them from ideas. Again, very similar to Freud's explorations of the role of the recognition of the reality as an important part of the mental functioning (Freud, 1911).

Clearly distinguishing the mind of a human from the mind of an animal, Uznadze also did not believe in the value of observations of animal behaviour with their generalization to human behaviour. That view made Uznadze a subject of criticism in times when the whole science was based on the ideas of Pavlov, who based conclusions about human physiology from studies on dogs. His study was concerned with the personality as an integral factor of mental activity, and for that he criticized 'bourgeois' science, dealing with studies of separate mental functions. The subject of the personality should not be interpreted based on the individual mental functions, quite the opposite – "all mental functions must be interpreted on the basis of the subject himself" (p. 205).

In 1977, Prangishvili summarized the contribution made by Uznadze who

> demonstrated theoretically and experimentally that unconscious mental activity is a constituent element in any act of human behaviour. Its role is especially great in the creative processes that manifest themselves in the development of science, the arts and language. In addition, the set theory made it possible to gain deeper knowledge about the causes of a number of diseases.
> (Prangishvili, 1977, p. 13)

That text was written before the International Symposium on the Problem of Unconscious in 1978, where multiple discussions of the theory of set were presented, and the name of Uznadze was free from ideological criticism. A Symposium that was a result of Filipp Bassin's enormous effort in re-setting the attitude towards the unconscious in Soviet academia.

## Filipp Bassin, the unconscious, and other activity

I have already described how Filipp Bassin set out an example of quasi-criticism being used as a way to inform the reader about 'prohibited' ideas, especially in his 'ground-breaking' book on the unconscious. He was remembered by his disciples as an enthusiast of undercover psychoanalysis (Shoshin, 1992; Arnold, 1999), that he moved to Moscow to become a member of psychoanalytic society, but arrived a little too late as the ideological campaign against it was in bloom.

Born in 1905 in Kharkiv, into a Jewish family, Filipp Bassin studied medicine and after graduation in 1931 worked as a researcher in the Kharkiv Psychoneurological Academy and an assistant in the Department of Psychopathology in the All-Ukrainian Psychoneurological Academy.[7] There he worked together with Luria and other members of the Vygotsky Circle. In 1936 he moved to Moscow to work in the All-Union Institute of Experimental Medicine, which after 1945 was transformed into the Institute of Neurology AMS USSR (Karpenko, 2005, pp. 39–40). During 1942–1943 he was in Kisegach as a head of the electroencephalography room.[8]

Like many scientists of that time who initially worked in the field of psychology or psychiatry, Bassin had to change his scientific interests, shifting from a medical career to studies in neurophysiology. His first dissertation was dedicated to the study of the alteration of word meanings in schizophrenia and was made under the influence of Vygotsky's work on schizophrenia (Yasnitsky, 2015). It was completed in 1935.[9] In Zeigarnik's monograph I found a brief mention of Bassin's idea that in schizophrenia we observe the appearance of something called a 'verbal tumour', with reference to this dissertation. However, everywhere in the archives it is indicated as a manuscript, and perhaps was never printed.

His second dissertation for the doctorate degree was dedicated to the analysis of EEG changes in the brain after craniocerebral damages and based on the research he did during WWII in Kisegach. Electroencephalography of brain damages could have been a good cover for psychological research in this time of persecution, but could also have been his genuine interest, not contradictory to his interest in psychoanalysis. Archival documents around the doctoral thesis defence contain a lot of interesting details. His reviewer, Professor M. N. Livanov[10] notices that one of the weaknesses of the work is Bassin's "unacceptably 'free' uses of the physiological and physical terminology" and contains several wrong physiological conclusions.[11] The reviewer also notices a 'heavy' style of writing, so "to read the work required significant psychic exertion". To me, that indicates the emergence of the specific scientific style of writing, that Bassin adopted to confuse his readers.

Opponents to his defence were P. K. Anokhin, S. A. Sarkisov[12] and N. I. Grashchenkov.[13][14] Grashchenkov noted that the main strength of Bassin's work was that it is a fundamental study of the electric activity of the brain after injuries,[15] never done before. Sarkisov[16] agrees with the critique that Bassin gives of Western studies of EEG for rather linear connections of electric activity and functions. Anokhin[17] gives overall a very positive review. The reviewer N. A. Bernstein[18][19] highlights that Bassin argues rightly that study of the electric activity of brain has its limitations due to the impossibility of equating electric activity of the neurons only to oscillations of the machine.

There is an important detail – all reviewers mentioned that Bassin referenced Pavlov in the research – a required code word for Bassin to be accepted and a signature of the ideological complexity of times. Also, all the reviewers pointed that the formulations Bassin presented were sometimes too long and too complicated, so the reader can understand their meaning only after re-reading them several times. This style of writing, with its pseudo-scientific complexity, was another signature of the ideological complexity of times. That style was both an attempt to create a 'clever' impression and to confuse someone outside academia, for example a party/police member, who would not be able to understand it and hence not able to attack it.

Bassin's doctorate dissertation on the EEG study could have been published as a book. All opponents mention this in their reviews, quite rightly expecting to see their corrections acknowledged in the published monograph. However, this publication never happened. Instead, Bassin published the monograph dedicated to the problem of the unconscious.

The history of Bassin's publications before he received his doctorate degree in 1957 and after is strikingly different[20]:

1932–1933 Works on professional orientation, on the collective tests;
1935 dissertation on the question of the alteration in word meaning in schizophrenia;
1937–1940 Three publications, on the functional approach in the brain studies and the rehabilitation of functions after brain injuries;
1944–1957 Around 20 publications, including 12 articles on electro-encephalography and localizations, the rest is miscellaneous;
1957 – Dissertation on the EEG;
1958–1960 12 publications on the question of Freudism, scientific discussion on the unconscious, the French school of psychosomatic medicine.[21]

We can see that in two years between 1958 and 1960 he published the same number of articles as in the previous 13. Perhaps Bassin even wrote them over the previous years but had no way to publish them until the right time. It might be also, that after getting a degree and obtaining a position in academia he felt more protected and so had more freedom to research what he was interested in all these years. It is difficult to imagine that in the years 1930–1950 he could get a degree by defending a dissertation on Freud. Either way this number of publications is indicative of his commitment to psychoanalytic theory, which was never lost or abandoned by him.

Perhaps, not surprisingly, his colleagues Shoshin (1992) remembers Bassin as an undercover agent whose activity helped to protect psychological ideas as well as real people during times of ideological purges in science. Kozulin (1984) argues the same, through Bassin psychoanalytic theory did not disappear completely between 1930 and 1980, so when after the fall of the Soviet Union the time to 'rehabilitate' psychoanalysis came, it was possible to do so. "Bassin was successful in demonstrating that the problem of the unconscious is much wider than its psychoanalytic interpretation – which implied that Soviet psychologists could approach this problem without being compromised by a liaison with Freud's doctrine" (Kozulin, 1989, p. 241).

As a result of that work on rehabilitation of Freud, in 1968 in Moscow his book *The Problem of the Unconscious* (published with 10,000 copies) appeared in stores and, according to Shoshin (1992) almost immediately was sold out. The freedom to mention Freud's name was a crucial turn in psychological science in the USSR and was very much in tune with the spirit of 1968. "The joy of using prohibited words should be balanced by a necessary dosage of ostentatious scepticism" (Shoshin, 1992). Shoshin argues that to rehabilitate repressed psychoanalysis in the USSR was a long-lasting goal of Bassin. "When he became a graduated psychiatrist, he mastered the psychoanalytic method, was an ardent supporter of Freud's theory, admired his charismatic personality" (Shoshin, 1992). His move to Moscow coincided with the period of existence of the Moscow Psychoanalytic Society run by Alexander Luria, with whom he had worked already in Kharkiv. Bassin hoped to realize his analytical talent, but the changes of the mid-1930s made it impossible to mention Freud's name and anything related to it (Shoshin, 1992). In the political context of that time, Bassin possessed the most useful ability – he spoke the language of authorities, the Marx-Lenin rhetoric that provided him and his circle with a shield against defenestration and helped to keep his research going. After defending his second dissertation in 1957, Bassin had the time and academic freedom to dedicate himself to the topic he has always been interested in, the problem of the unconscious (Shoshin, 1992). His monograph collected a wide range of names and views on the problem of the unconscious in the West, and for an ordinary doctor or scholar, his book could be the only source to get to know them. "The book made a splash in the cultural centres of the USSR" (Shoshin, 1992). The reference Bassin made in his book to work of Dmitry Uznadze and the theory of set opened the possibility for further expansion of studies of the unconscious. A combined effort of Moscow and Tbilisi resulted in the International Symposium on the Unconscious in 1979 with several delegations of international participants. Among them were significant names such as Jacobson and in the French group Andre Green and Didier Anzieu. Three volumes of materials were prepared and edited by Bassin to be published before the beginning of the Symposium, each of them around 300 pages.

### Bassin's return to Freud

In 1960, *Soviet Review* published a translation of Bassin's article 'A Debate on Freudism' [*Freidizm v svete sovremennykh nauchnykh diskussii*] that was originally published in *Voprosy Psikhologii* in 1958.[22] A key point for reopening of the discussion of Freud's work is the fact that, in 1954, *The Project for a Scientific Psychology* (1895) had been published for the first time. For Bassin, *The Project* offers the reason for reconsideration of psychoanalytic theory development. As he reasonably points out, "Freud's methodological views in this period are reflected in his characteristic conviction that inasmuch as we know little about the physiological mechanisms of the brain, psychological theory must be elaborated independently of physiology" (Bassin, 1960, p. 4). Perhaps at this point the reader will notice, with curiosity, the fact that the Soviet scientist is aware of the publication of the Freud's *Project* and apparently read it as well, despite the 'eradication' and 'ban' of Freud.

Interestingly enough, *The Project* played an important role in the return to Freud for Lacan and for Derrida. Can we consider that Soviet academics had their own 'return' to Freud? In 1958, the resonance of the Pavlov Session and the need to keep loyal to reflexology was still present, and psychology was still under ideological pressure. That itself could be enough for Bassin to be obliged to link Freud to physiology. However, what if the interest in physiology was genuine and caused the emergence of original findings?

Bassin's work clearly demonstrates his shift away from simplistic brain localization in favour of exploring interconnections and regulatory systems within physiology. Like his contemporaries, psychophysiologists N. Bernstein and P. Anokhin, he sought to understand how systems interact rather than pinpointing exact functional locations. By this time, the research by Anokhin and Luria had already highlighted the brain's remarkable adaptability, showing that if a brain centre responsible for a function such as speech or movement were damaged, rehabilitation could enable the creation of new centres to take over the lost function. Drawing on the theories of functional systems and the set, Bassin argued that Soviet physiology should revisit Freud's abandoned exploration of the unconscious, emphasizing its critical role and the need for scientific study. While this perspective may have been partly tailored to address the political sensitivities of the Party, whose influence loomed in the background, it also represented a genuine question for Bassin: how to approach Freud's ideas anew, integrating recent physiological insights and experimental methods.

If we set aside general points of criticism, in this article, Freud interests Bassin for the idea of energy circulation in pathological states: "emotional experience which produces an urge to definite action possesses a store of energy that tries to manifest itself in behaviour. Suppressed, this energy can provoke hysterical symptoms" (Bassin, 1960, p. 5). Of course, Freud did not succeed in studying this energy properly, e.g., physiologically, says Bassin, due to the limited scientific knowledge of his times. Thus, experimental investigation of supressed impulses in Freud's work is absent (p. 10), but it doesn't mean for Bassin that it is impossible. As an example of a proper experimental study of the influence of supressed impulses he brings the Zeigarnik effect (p. 11).

### Bassin's unconscious

If Bassin was interested in energy circulation and the possibility of capturing the unconscious by experimental methods, how much of an alternative did his theory pose to the Freudian unconscious? This section explores various ways in which Bassin approached the unconscious, summarized in his monograph titled *The Problem of the Unconscious* [*Problema bessoznatel'nogo*], published in 1968.

The total volume of his work is 460 pages, divided into six chapters. The first chapter is methodological. The second offers the history of the 'unconscious' before psychoanalysis and psychosomatic medicine. The third offers a review of Freud's biography and psychoanalytic ideas. The fourth is dedicated to the non-conscious forms of the psyche and higher nervous activity in the light of the theory of biological regulation and the theory of set. The fifth chapter is concerned with the role of non-conscious higher nervous activity in the regulation of psychophysiological activity and behaviour. The sixth chapter presents conclusions and perspectives on the problem of the unconscious.

When Bassin reviews existing opinions on Freud's ideas, his knowledge of international events, critique and polemics in the psychoanalytic field appears to be very detailed. He is aware of the latest conferences in the West and published discussions around psychoanalysis (Bassin, 1968, pp. 79–85). This seems to resolve the question of the isolation of Soviet scientists, which if it existed would have made it impossible for Bassin to know so much about the psychoanalytic field. Thus, from the introduction, Bassin's interest in psychoanalysis was apparent. However, on what level was he engaged with psychoanalytic ideas and how deep was his understanding of Freud?

While psychoanalysis as a clinical method and social theory raises many questions and doubts (p. 90) for Bassin, the psychological side and the theory of the unconscious remains outside criticism. He recognizes an important element of the Freudian theory of the unconscious – derivates of the repressed material – arguing that the destiny of those 'dissociated elements' and their role and pathologizing impact on conscious psychic activity is something to be studied (p. 93). Those 'dissociated elements' or the derivates of the repressed are crucial for the psychoanalytic notion of the unconscious because their presence distinguishes between the unconscious understood as 'non-conscious' and the Freudian unconscious.

For Bassin, the point of agreement with psychoanalysis is the talking cure, or release of symptoms by the realization of unconscious material, in other words by transfer of unconscious material into consciousness (p. 93). Just a simple realization, though, is not enough. He suggests building on Uznadze's theory to enhance the understanding of how exactly the therapeutic effect must be achieved: the new presentation (realized idea) should be included in the current 'set' system or cause the appearance of the new 'set' and direct the attitude of the person towards reality (p.95). Otherwise, argues Bassin, it will stay just a realization and will not influence the further activity of the person. Whether he was aware of this or not, the idea of the inclusion of the unconscious idea into the current situation of life and change of attitude towards reality was one of the key points of Freudian technique, which Freud described in *Remembering, Repeating and Working Through* (1914). But even if this was not a hidden reference, Bassin shows quite a deep understanding of Freudian psychic mechanisms.

Cesare Musatti concludes the same in his response to Bassin's article:

> The words used by F.V. Bassin, criticizing the simplified way of interpreting the effect of recovery, which came as a result of the fact that the repressed impulses rise to the level of consciousness, almost repeat the words written by Freud in 1914 on this subject in the article 'Erinnern, Wiederholen und Durcharbeiten', in which Freud sets out the modifications already achieved at that time by the technique of analysis, establishing more precisely and concretely the relationship between the repressed impulses and the patient's personality as a whole.
> 
> (Mussatti in Bassin, 1968, p. 396)

The full text (200 pages) of exchanges between Bassin's and Musatti was published as an additional chapter of Bassin's monograph. Overall, Musatti presents important points of the misunderstanding of the critique towards Freud written by Bassin. For Musatti, acknowledged with Freud, it is apparent that Bassin criticizes Freud by using Freud's own words from his later period to address issues in his ideas from the earlier period. That detail, however, is only visible to the reader knowledgeable about Freudian ideas. For someone who never read Freud – for example Party authorities – this paradox stayed invisible.

Perhaps for that reason, later psychologists from the 1990s blindly criticized psychoanalysis following their older colleagues' 'critique' without understanding it. This paradox is captured in the paper of the former pupil of Bassin, Olga Arnold:

> My beloved professor was so proficient in the Aesopian language, was such a skilful diplomat that he could fool not only limited censors from science but even inexperienced psychologists! For the new generation of scientists, who have long, in English terms, called a spade a spade, this is even more difficult to understand, just as many Western experts on the unconscious cannot understand it.
> 
> (Arnold, 1999, p. 101)

Let's return to our reading. Something else becomes apparent from the exchange between Bassin and Musatti. While Musatti addresses Bassin's incompetence in criticising Freud for his early ideas, which were later revised and rethought by him and his followers, Bassin emphasizes, in his response, that the Soviet critique of psychoanalysis is not situated on the level of the content of the theory. Psychoanalysis, says Bassin, is mostly criticized for its incompatibility with the direction of communism and its 'reactionary' nature as he names it. Psychoanalysis puts too much weight on the subject in reasoning and helps capitalist society to avoid responsibility for exploitation and the mental state of people (Bassin, 1968, p. 406).

This discussion raises the question of whether it would it be possible in other circumstances to publish Musatti in the Soviet Union. Probably not or most likely not, as he was a Western psychoanalyst and hence lived and practiced 'anti-Soviet ideas'. What if Bassin organized these polemics precisely for that reason? As with other examples I have given, it seems that although Bassin's account of psychoanalysis was presented as criticism, it functioned to make psychoanalysis available for the Soviet reader. His thinking about psychoanalysis, his clarification of Freud's ideas stayed available for the reader who was interested to know. And if Yurchak was right and citizens in the 1960s actively employed authoritarian discourse, for them to recognize and to decode this strategy of Bassin was quite simple. Nor surprisingly then, as Olga Arnold remembers,[23] in the 1970s almost everyone practiced or attempted to practice psychoanalysis in the psychiatric hospital where she was undergoing her post-university placement. According to her, psychoanalysis was fused with other methods, so it would be more precise to say it was a psychoanalytically informed practice. Overall, interest and discussion around psychoanalysis was lively and so the demand for psychoanalytic texts would have been significant. While, at least in the Public Library in Leningrad, in the 1970s to obtain a copy of Freud was not very complicated, but still required a special pass,[24] the discussion about Freudian core concepts was available for the reader of Musatti and Bassin's polemics without any restriction.

### The Soviet response to the problem of the unconscious

Further on in the monograph we find a critical review of Freud and psychosomatic medicine, in which he shows a good knowledge of the ideas of Abraham, Ferenczi and Klein – again, impressive given the 'ban' or 'abandonment' of psychoanalysis and 'turn' to Pavlov (Bassin, 1968, pp. 97–120). The critique's main points against Freud for Bassin are the insufficient physiological ground for the theory of the unconscious. This is how he brings the reader to the main argument – the Soviet view on the problem of the unconscious (p. 123).

Bassin emphasizes many times that it is important to study the unconscious and that Soviet science has made some progress towards it. However, it is crucial for us to understand what kind of unconscious it was and what use Soviet studies of the unconscious can be for psychoanalytic theory today. If we ignore the familiar criticism that Freud failed to find physiological ground for his theories, and therefore that they are not scientific, and continue reading, an interesting horizon opens up. It looks like Bassin presents an account of the Freudian unconscious, whether intentionally or not, supporting his summary by evidence gained in the laboratories of Soviet physiologists. "A Freudian unconscious about to be proved by Soviet physiologists!" – that would be a great headline in *Pravda*.

Bassin begins with the definition, so the reader can orientate to his object of study, but very soon he puts the reader into the maze. Let's follow him to untangle the 'Soviet' notion of the unconscious.

Bassin distinguishes non-conscious and unconscious activity, wakefulness and consciousness. For him there is no need to prove that mental being is supported by higher nervous system activity, although we cannot reduce the unconscious to the non-conscious processes of the nervous system. Similarly, the state of wakefulness should not be equated to consciousness. This crystalized the aim of his study: it is 'non-conscious forms of psychic activity' rather than 'non-conscious forms of higher nervous activity' (p. 131). However, 'the non-conscious forms of psychic activity' will not stay for long in Bassin's vocabulary. Thirty pages later Bassin will notice that most of the higher nervous activity and hence psychic activity is non-conscious anyway, and this term does not represent accurately the real object of his study, but there is no other term found yet, and "it is no longer possible not to have a corresponding concept at all" ( p. 167). And then he suggests, there is a suitable word, although with the bad stigma, as it is related to psychoanalysis. Despite this stigma, he will use the term unconscious further in his text but will put it into commas to emphasize that the term is taken from psychoanalysis but not. In other words, Bassin says: we have alternative terms in our vocabulary to study the unconscious, but really these terms do not represent what we want to study, and hence we will use the term from psychoanalysis – although we don't support psychoanalytic ideas in Soviet Union. This strategy, I'll put in Freud's words,

> reminded one vividly of the defence put forward by the man who was charged by one of his neighbours with having given him back a borrowed kettle in a damaged condition. The defendant asserted first, that he had given it back undamaged; secondly, that the kettle had a hole in it when he borrowed it; and thirdly, that he had never borrowed a kettle from his neighbour at all.
>
> (Freud, 1900, p. 119)

After Bassin 'borrowed the kettle', he proceeded to explain what kind of 'unconscious' was studied. If consciousness should be understood not only as a state of wakefulness, then the 'unconscious' is not just non-conscious. The traditional understanding of consciousness in Soviet psychology is wider and rooted in the Marxist philosophy highlighting that human consciousness and personality develop through practical engagement with the world. It includes the subject who can participate in the perception of reality and develop a specific relation to it (p. 126). Consciousness thus becomes very much connected with the activity (*deiatel'nost*) – purposeful interaction of a subject with the world, through which the subject transforms both their environment and themselves – of the subject and represents his/her system of motives and values (p. 126). However, Bassin doesn't fully believe in the total consciousness and clear activity. While our active subject participates in the state of wakefulness, the notion of consciousness does not cover moments when the subject can recognize certain states but does not perceive them as subjective states (p. 161). Bassin calls these states 'split off' (*otscheplenie*) and defines them as the main object of interest, as they are exactly non-conscious forms of the higher nervous activity indicating the existence of the 'unconscious' (p. 169).

This bit of Bassin's thinking echoes the limitations of consciousness that are also described by Freud. While we can recognize and direct our active attention to psychic 'events' that appear in the field of our conscious, we are not in control of many of them, which appear as slips of the tongue, mistakes, and episodes of forgetfulness – parapraxes. They are exactly split-offs, psychic events of the kind that for Freud prove the existence of the unconscious not only as non-conscious material, but as an active part of the mind, being charged with its own agenda – wishes and drives, being formed according to its own 'unconscious' logic, etc. (Freud, 1915). Bassin's definition of the 'split off' states are wider and include more than parapraxes.

To understand it better, let's step out of Bassin's monograph for a moment. In his speech at the All-Union Conference dedicated to the Philosophical Problems of the Higher Nervous Activity in 1963, he pointed out several problems, including the period of silence in research on the unconscious due to the political charge towards psychoanalysis and the gap this created in the understanding of the unconscious activity of the mind. One of the methodological problems, however, is that Soviet studies are engaged with Marxist ideas, where consciousness and activity are interrelated, and therefore the Soviet study of the mind is concerned with both predominantly. Behind the consciousness, however, Bassin suggests noticing the 'active attitude towards reality'. In other words, Bassin says that we have a subject (individual) whose perception of reality is not based on reflection but caused by the complex of internal reasons – motives, needs, interests – which, in their turn are based on the existence of the body and physiological processes. Bassin gives a notion of consciousness as being only a part of mental activity, and highlights that we cannot equate consciousness to the mind.

Furthermore, Bassin brings in Uznadze as a representative of the Soviet studies of the unconscious, whose experimental work proved the existence of such internal reasons and included them in his notion of the set. As we know, Uznadze was not the most favoured figure, so Bassin's rhetoric of bringing the theory of set was again the 'kettle technique'. He points out that Uznadze's set is a totally unconscious structure without the possibility of an individual becoming aware of it. That, says Bassin, makes Uznadze's theory very close to the Freudian idea of the unconscious (Bassin, 1963, p. 469) and therefore must be rejected. Bassin writes 'we decline' (*my otkloniaem*) it and refuse to accept the fully unconscious status of the set, while at the same time he suggests using the notion of the set as useful for further explanation of unconscious psychic activity.

Back to the monograph. Bassin compares the set to the notion of the 'dynamic stereotype' by Pavlov. The difference between them is that the set is regulated by subjective value, while dynamic stereotype reactions are established randomly. Importantly, we see how the category of *meaning* is included in the notion of 'the set' while 'dynamic stereotype' is constructed without it. To break the dynamic stereotype a person just needs to establish a new series of reactions, while the change of 'set' requires a shift in meaning (Bassin, 1968, pp. 215–216). Thus, it is not just enough, as in the CBT approach to foster a habit of 'healthy' behaviour by the repetition of sequences of new actions and the establishment of new dynamic stereotypes. In the case of the 'the set', a person needs to recognize *why* it is valuable and put it in accordance with not only conscious, but also the unconscious.

This brings us to the next point of discussion, important for Bassin – the status of affects in the unconscious. He is curious and wants to understand the paradox of unconscious affect and what psychological and physiological consequences this unconscious affect has on the whole system of the psyche. And if this unconscious affect transforms into the fixed system of the tendencies of regulation, or the system of the set. Basically, this suggests that the transformation of affect can lead to the forming of the set. He references Anokhin's theory of emotions (p. 219) as regulators of activity, playing a crucial role in his theory of the functional system and serving as feedback correcting activity. He then adds that psychoanalysis never really studied this regulatory function of emotions (p. 218).

For Bassin, when the affect is put into the unconscious, it does not disappear but creates the basis for action [activity]. The affect in the unconscious transforms subjective values for certain actions and attachments – this is the creation of the set. Therefore the set is created by affective charge:

> When we stop fixing our attention on a certain emotion, for example, on the feeling of love, the emotion from this, of course, does not disappear. But in what form, in what sense is it preserved? It persists in the sense that once it has arisen, it rearranges in a certain way the system of our behaviour, creates (regardless of whether it is realized at the moment or not) a certain direction of our actions, the desire to react in a certain way,

the preference of some actions and avoidance of others. In a word, it creates what is called a certain 'set' not only in psychology but also in everyday speech. It is in this and only in this sense that we can say that our feelings persist in us, despite the fact that the phenomena to which our attention is riveted, the contents of our conscious experiences are constantly changing. Our affects and strivings persist in us in the form of attitudes. The paradoxical idea of 'repressed', that is, feelings experienced subjectively, should be refined, at best, as an attempt to express very complex facts without the help of rigorous scientific concepts especially developed for this.

(footnote, p. 220)

Therefore, when we replace the concept of 'repressed affect' with the concept of 'unconscious set', we clarify the really existing scheme of functional relations.

Indeed, since Freud's shift from the cathartic method to the talking cure the focus has been on language and insights, rather than experiencing things affectively. There is, however, no contradiction with psychoanalysis in this regard: our affects persist in the mind, where they are included in the circulation of libidinal energy and presentations. As Freud emphasizes, in fact,

> three such vicissitudes are possible: either the affect remains, wholly or in part, as it is; or it is transformed into a qualitatively different quota of affect, above all into anxiety; or it is suppressed, i.e. it is prevented from developing at all.
>
> (Freud, 1915 p. 178)

Thus, this is another example of a 'critique' being in fact a discussion of Freud's idea. So the question remains unanswered: was there anything Soviet added to the idea of the unconscious, after all? My answer is no – at the core, the understanding of the unconscious is conceptually no different in Freud's and Bassin's writing. What is new in the Soviet approach to the unconscious is the attempt to include physiological studies into its scope and develop a sort of experimental approach to study the unconscious. As we've seen in the chapters dedicated to Zeigarnik and Luria, these two specifics constituted their research as well.

It appears Bassin's aim was to bring psychoanalytic ideas into the academic discussions of the times. His further activity solidified around publishing, translations and establishing contacts with international colleagues.

In 1976, Bassin prepared for publication and edited the book on the Marxist critique of Freudism by Catherine Clément, Pierre Bruno and Lucien Sève, *Pour une critique marxiste de la théorie psychanalytique* (1973). In the preface he discusses the idea that psychoanalysis is not a united discipline, there are many different schools – in a way he is splitting psychoanalysis away from Freud's name. He notes the value of Freud's ideas as rethought by Lacan, who is problematic himself, but worthy of discussion.[25] One of the notes I found important in Bassin's introduction to this volume is the argument that the theoretical value of some of the ideas of psychoanalysis by Marxist thinkers should not necessarily lead to psychomarxism (1976, p. 31). Partial appreciation of psychoanalytic ideas and critical thinking, as well as awareness of the capacity of psychoanalysis to be self-critical, prepared a path for the gradual return of psychoanalysis in the late 1970s. Another idea Bassin offers in his preface is that contemporary psychology should rethink core psychoanalytic concepts like 'ego defences', 'Oedipus complex' etc. accordingly to the socio-political context to find a place for them in studies of the mind (p. 39).

Bassin was one of the main organizers the International Symposium on the Unconscious that took place in Tbilisi in 1979. He also organized the publication of the four volumes of the symposium, that will be discussed in the next part of this chapter.

After the fall of the Soviet Union, within a relatively free society where psychoanalysis was 'rehabilitated' by Yeltsin's decree, together with Prof Yaroshevsky in 1991 Bassin edited and published Freud's *Lectures on Psychoanalysis [Vvedeniie v Psikhoanaliz. Lekcii]* (Bassin and Yaroshevsky, 1991).

I am sure all these publications and events are only a small, visible part of Bassin's activity, and with further research focused on his life, it will be possible to obtain more evidence of his huge contribution. Despite appearing to criticise Freud in each of his published works, Bassin did much to promote Freud's ideas and make them available to the public. 'Decline and refuse, but at the same time actively engage with the topic' – that, in short, seems like a motto for the Bassin's approach that helped him to navigate in keeping psychoanalysis 'alive' for 50 years of the Soviet 'ban'.

## Between Moscow and Tbilisi: The Symposium on the Unconscious, 1979

Twenty years after the Freud Session, an event occurred that has not slipped the attention of anyone who has researched the history of psychoanalysis in Soviet times, the 1979 Tbilisi Symposium on the Unconscious.

It is difficult to say something new when so many researchers have already presented detailed accounts of its organization (Rotenberg, 2015; Mazin, 2018) and the meaning of the event for the rehabilitation of psychoanalysis (Miller, 1998; Angelini, 2008). In this section I am going to examine key papers from the four volumes of the symposium (Prangishvili, Sherozia and Bassin 1978a, 1978b, 1978c, 1985) that present a Soviet academic 'take' on it. As we will see, some of contributions genuinely engaged with Freud's ideas, some used the same 'kettle' technique as Bassin, and some genuinely criticized psychoanalysis. For what it's worth, each volume is around 700 pages of discussion on the unconscious.

## Volume I: 'Nature, Functions, and Methods of Study' of the unconscious

Volume 1 opens with a set of articles on the reality of the phenomena of the unconscious. As we know, Freud's 'proofs' of the existence of the unconscious are hypnotic states, slips of the tongue and various 'mistakes' that occur in everyday life, dreams, and symptoms. For the Soviet academics, the existence of the unconscious was 'proved' by a series of experiments on the set, done by Uznadze and his school. We may say that the relation between the notion of the unconscious and the notion of set is a political question, since the debate around it was not concerned with how exactly the study of the set engaged with the unconscious, but whether it was possible to 'trace' references to bourgeois idealistic psychology in there, or whether it was a 'pure' Soviet science.

The reasons for the gradual fading of interest in psychoanalysis since the 1920s are given in the preface to this volume through the shift that psychoanalytic theory underwent in general. Being primarily a clinical method, it received wide acceptance by clinicians in Russia. The expansion of psychoanalysis into a "doctrine of a philosophical and social kind" (Sherozia, 1978, p. 26) made it alien to the ideological stance of Soviet psychology and medicine. But what about the notion of the unconscious? It made a dialectical move from Freud's particular unconscious to the general notion of Uznadze's set.

The introductory article to the volume, written by one of the organizers of the symposium, Apollon Sherozia, in many aspects is a typical example of Soviet engagement with psychoanalysis. It contains a 'traditional' critique of Freud, combined with the original ideas that build on top of his theory. In my view this was a productive critique that offers certain solutions for the studies of the unconscious, that at the same time stays within the 'spirit' of psychoanalysis. However, the opposition to Freudian ideas was necessary and continuously reiterated through the text in the form of negation.

The first part of the article is dedicated to a criticism of Freud. In the best tradition established after 1958, Sherozia denies any connections with Freud's psychoanalysis but wishes to continue to explore the notion of the unconscious. So it was not only Bassin who negated psychoanalysis for the sake of bringing its ideas to the fore of the attention. Sherozia approaches Freud from the philosophy standpoint and finds it problematic that Freud does not know what the ontic status is of the unconscious and what various presentations turn into after being repressed from consciousness, hence the Freudian unconscious is a negative of the conscious (Sherozia, 1978, p. 38). The set, on the other hand, is a positive phenomenon, highlighting Sherozia. For someone not familiar with Freudian writings that kind of critique sounded convincing. While it is true that in the work *The Unconscious* (1915) Freud uses the particle 'no' much more than other words to describe the status and characteristics of the unconscious, he does affirm the unconscious as a phenomenon different from just the negative of the conscious. Unlikely Sherozia was not a good reader of Freud and overlooked this aspect in his work.

Sherozia goes further to identify specific aspects of the set and names them as such:

1. it is a special form (or a formation) of the psyche;
2. this special formation influences perception (Sherozia, 1978, p. 41);
3. the set is always a situation, which includes the drive and the object, as well as a form of relationship between them as determined by the drive.

For Uznadze, the set is an ultimate core construction of the person's being. It forms a 'special scope' of reality and without the participation of the set we cannot see any mental processes. The set forms a dimension of psychic reality (pp. 43–44).

This description brings the set closer to the unconscious phantasy, as formulated by Klein. While she recognizes, following Freud, libidinal drives being at the core of the unconscious, for her there is no impulse of the drive which is not experienced as an unconscious phantasy that includes objects or representation of certain kind of relations in attempt to make sense of these impulses:

> an activity of the mind that occurs on deep unconscious levels and accompanies every impulse experienced by the infant.... Phantasies – becoming more elaborate and referring to a wider variety of objects and situations – continue throughout development and accompany all activities; they never stop playing a great part in mental life.
> (Klein, 1959, p. 250)

Thus "for Klein, the drive is always mediated through unconscious phantasy, which is its psychical representation or manifestation ... the emphasis she places on phantasy suggests that we can't have any unmediated access to this aspect of our experience" (Allen and Ruti, 2019, p. 92).

The similarity between the set and unconscious phantasy becomes even clearer when Sherozia offers a critique of Soviet psychology of personality and especially of some of the statements of activity theory, where research is centred around the personality, and functions like thinking and perception are seen as dependent on it. He brings to the fore two formulas (Sherozia, 1978, p. 45): "external causes act through internal conditions" from S. D. Rubinstein, and "the internal (subject) acts through the external and thereby changes itself" from D. A. Leontiev. Both are summarized through the statement "it is not the mind that thinks, but a person". Sherozia's position is different: "the internal and the external interact in the subject only through the fundamental unity of its integrated systemic set", or to make it simpler, neither reality nor person dictate what is perceived or thought, it is the set – the structure that integrates experiences and mental functions.

An important elaboration Sherozia makes is that psychoanalysis focuses on the continuous split of the mind into unconscious and conscious processes, while from the position of the theory of set their interaction is seen through their phenomenological unity (pp. 51–52). He identifies two sub-structures of the unconscious: 1. the pre-conscious structure, or the set itself; 2. post-conscious unconscious experiences, like desires, memories, goals, thoughts etc. that become a material for dreams and can form various mental processes (p. 52). This division explains why and how certain mental material can be repressed[26] from consciousness and then be returned to it. For that we must accept the set as a primary unconscious structure, that can animate and regulate post-conscious unconscious mental material (p. 53). Such a division makes sense from the psychoanalytic perspective, if we include the question of the psychic (mental) structure in our discussion. Freud's classification of structures includes neurotic, psychotic, and perverse structures, all of which have their own sets of 'defences' that organize and structure mental processes. Some Lacanians add melancholic structure on top of this classification. For Klein, a similar formulation on the structure was made in terms paranoid-schizoid and depressive structures of unconscious phantasies. Sherozia's text, from that perspective, appears as a thoughtful account and an attempt to elaborate the idea of the unconscious, and shows that the level of engagement with psychoanalytic ideas in Soviet academia was quite substantial.

Overall, acceptance of the phenomena of the unconscious and its implications on the understanding of the work of mind of the individual appears to be common position amongst practitioners.

From the collections of papers in the first part of the Volume I we can outline several basic statements on the unconscious, that all authors agree with.

1  The unconscious is an integral structure of the mind

> Numerous psychological observations make us think that our state of mind in each individual case is not limited by what is represented in consciousness. Observations speak in favour of the fact that conscious and unconscious mental processes create a single integral structure within which our daily mental life proceeds.
> (Chkhartishvili, 1978, p. 103)

2  Activity is overdetermined by the unconscious

> According to Uznadze, the scope of the unconscious psyche is so wide that it underlies all human activity, both internal and external. The functions of the unconscious are not limited to what psychoanalysis says about them. Neither in behaviour, nor consciousness, nor in practical action, does anything happen that is not determined by the unconscious.
> (p. 107)

> In the experiments on mental activity, where the practical activity of an individual is studied, the unconscious fixed set can participate and influence how individuals categorize the stimuli, classify them to certain categories and the duration of the chosen reaction. The same kind of facts of the unconscious influence of the set were discovered in studies of sensorimotor activity.
>
> (Nadirashvili, 1978, p. 116)

Also it was discovered that the set influences intellectual activity (p. 117) and there is a social set (p. 118).

Thus, the idea of the unconscious was not alien to Soviet academia. One of the unique features of the Soviet academic approach to the unconscious, apparent from this volume, is methodology. All the discoveries above were observed experimentally. While there is not much indication of how these experiments were conducted, we can suggest that experimental situations included various tasks offered to participants – most likely patients in the hospital or day clinic – their responses measured and documented. Many of them are discussed in Uznadze's (1966) monograph, where participants are offered to hold and compare objects of various shapes and weights, fill gaps in texts to reconstruct stories, etc. It is possible to imagine, however, that the emphasis on the experimental nature of theoretical conclusions was a necessity rather than a choice in the climate of Pavlov dominance over methods in psychology.

The second part of Volume I, represented mainly by the foreign participants from France and America, was dedicated to the history and evolution of the notion of the unconscious in psychoanalysis and its schools. Most of articles published in this volume are in French, English and German. On the one hand, that left them inaccessible for a wider audience, who might not have the knowledge of foreign languages. On the other hand, the fact that all these authors were published and were accessible for those who can read them, was a great achievement of Bassin and his colleagues. Among participants in the second part of the volume were such names as: Louis Althusser, Leon Chertok, Andre Green, Catrin Clement, Didieu Anzieu, Jean Paul Valabrega, Tomas F. Main, and Cesare Musatti. There were also articles by Soviet authors N. Avtonomova and L. Filippov about the structural psychoanalysis of Lacan. In the context of that times, this was another clever achievement of Bassin in making these authors available to the general public without a special pass to the library. Since they all were published as materials of the Soviet conference, they would not be considered as foreign publications and would be stored on open shelves.

The third part of the volume is concerned with the neurophysiology of the unconscious and presented by a mix of foreign and Soviet authors. The way some experiments were conducted indicated forces counter to the oppression of psychoanalysis; rather, it showed that studies of the unconscious were perhaps fashionable and spread beyond followers of Freud. For example, in one very curious paper, the collective of physiologists who studied the neurophysiological mechanism of drives stressed the importance of the Freudian idea of drives. To study the unconscious component of drives, the authors conducted a series of experiments ... with cats[27] (Sudakov and Kotov, 1978, p. 596). With all seriousness, they put Freud's *Three Essays on the Theory of Sexuality* (published in Russian in 1924) in the references.

There were more serious studies in this section as well, regarding the psychological defence mechanisms, emotional regulation, various experimental studies of the set and even endocrine mechanisms of regulation of unconscious stages of motivation development. I found especially interesting the paper by the American contributor, psychoanalyst Howard Shevrin, 'Neuropsychological Correlates of Psychodynamic Unconscious Processes' (Shevrin, 1978, p. 676–691), which offered neuropsychological evidence in support of the psychoanalytic assumption of the dynamic unconscious.

That bridge between neuropsychology and studies of the unconscious included in this volume could be not only curtseying to authorities, who aimed to keep the science clear of idealistic concepts. It could be an attempt to address the wide field of practitioners, who grew up conditioned to Pavlov's physiology and neuropsychological language.

## Volume II: 'Dreams, Clinic, Creativity'

Like the previous volume, Volume II contained papers in English, German, French and Russian that varied from serious studies to papers where the attempt was more valuable than the result. The preface to this volume removes any doubt about the level of understanding of psychoanalysis and accessibility of the psychoanalytic literature for Bassin, Prangishvili and Sherozia – the collective of editors and organizers of the Symposium.

> It is well known that this problem of the 'specific language' of the unconscious holds an important place in the psychoanalytic literature. It is rooted in Freud's early works which, for the first time, pointed to the existence of regular links between the activity of the unconscious and specific forms of conscious language production (slips of the tongue, slips of the pen, jokes, etc.). Subsequently this idea was considerably broadened due to its use in psychosomatic medicine (the viewing of certain diseases and clinical syndromes as symbolic 'body language' that gives expression to unconscious forms of mental activity or emotional states which, for some reason or other, are deprived of an opportunity of being expressed in behavioural acts and normal intercourse). Ultimately, in recent years attempts have been made – mainly as a result of Lacan's work – at further deepening the idea of the relation of the unconscious with language. These attempts are made under the modest slogan 'Back to Freud'.[28]
>
> (Prangishvili, Sherozia and Bassin, 1978b, p. 23)

This is only an extract of what was a thoughtful account of Lacan's 'return to Freud' and the status of language in psychoanalysis.[29] Again, this confirms that the engagement with psychoanalytic theory among at least the collective of editors of these volumes was not superficial. As we will see from the next part, the presence of Lacan's thought and his school gave rise to the new generation of followers of psychoanalysis, like Victor Mazin. The role of Bassin in promoting ideas of psychoanalysis and bringing various authors to be available to reader is quite apparent.

### Volume III: 'Cognition, Communication, Personality'

Volume III fully expanded the exploration of the unconscious and cognition, the role of language in the formation of thinking, intellect and information theory, and the role of the unconscious in developing personality. There is a special section on the unconscious, speech, and language highlighting papers by Roman Jacobson and Serge Leclaire. There is a stand-alone paper by Tavistock psychoanalyst B. Barnett on Balint Groups. The final part again returned to the question of the methods of study of the unconscious.

In the preface, the editors stress that despite the previous simplified views on the participation of the unconscious only at the level of 'elementary' mind, such as stereotyped activity and automatisms, it is now clear that

> the understanding of the irremovable presence of the unconscious in everything that is reflected in man's mental life as an expression of the highest forms of its organisation has largely altered our habitual notions of the very essence of these forms, and hence of the nature of mental life as a whole.
> (Prangishvili, Sherozia and Bassin, 1978c, p. 24)

Once again, this statement shows that at least Bassin's view on the nature of the mind was deeply anchored in the notion of the unconscious. Further on in the preface we find another fundamental idea that replicates an aspect of Freud's work:

> One can 'become conscious' – implying at least a developed form of the process – of only what 'has been named' or designated.... When formalised supraindividual objective 'meanings' become more or less closely superimposed on the uncommunicable 'significances' that gave them rise.... What is ... not being 'named', can exist as a psychological reality only in the form of the mental unconscious.
> (p. 25)

Perhaps, the clearest position on the place of the unconscious in the theory of personality is formulated in the paper by Apollon Sherozia, a Georgian philosopher and psychologist, who was one of the co-organizers of the Symposium. He sees the mind "not only as constituting a definite system of reflection or that of experiences but also as a definite system of relations" (p. 384). For him neither a theory of the unconscious nor a theory of consciousness will work without consideration of the dynamic relations between them, that in their turn organizes the system of the relations of the individual. It is important to note, that by relations here is understood not the relationships between two people, but the link, the connection, the reaction, of the mind of the individual to the object of external reality, including other people, and towards objects in the internal reality. They act for Sherozia as a whole, "functioning under a bilaterally mediated relationship through the initial psychophysiological unity of man, consciousness and the unconscious mind and constituting the basis of properly psychological characteristics of his personality over the entire range of its fundamental relations" (p. 386). That formulation is close to object relations theory, as formulated by Klein, who brings to the fore the notion of the internal objects, or partial objects, that populate the unconscious phantasy and therefore constitute the overall relationship of the individual towards themselves, others and the world.

## *Volume IV 'Results of the Discussion'*

Volume IV was published in the aftermath of the Symposium in 1985 and collected reflections of participants. An assessment of the impact of the Symposium we find in an article by Shoshin, a colleague of Bassin's whom we encountered earlier in this chapter. Shoshin summarizes the exit out of the struggle with the 'unconscious' that started in 1958.

The main question Shoshin discusses is how to conceptualize the unconscious. He points, rightly, to the fact that among participants of the Tbilisi Symposium there were some quite varied understandings of the unconscious. These he divided into three categories:

1   as psyche minus consciousness;
2   as a set of psychological phenomena and activities of which the subject is unaware; and
3   as a specific, positively defined component of the psyche.

The unconscious number 3 is a Freudian unconscious, and after a short discussion Shoshin concludes that this is the most fruitful way to conceptualize the unconscious and therefore it should be chosen by Soviet researchers (Shoshin, 1985, p. 171).

A detail that caught my attention while reading through the three volumes is the rarity of any critique of Freud of the kind that would have been formulated in the 1930s and 1950s. Moreover, the papers are picking up from where Freud reached his limit. This is what I suggest calling a Soviet return to

Freud – a productive elaboration of Freud's ideas, situated in Soviet circumstances. Not only was the Symposium a significant event, but it also marked the end of the era of criticism of Freud and opened doors for even more open discussion about psychoanalysis. For the new generation of academics, the materials of the Symposium became a collection of rare texts. But also, I think, the material of the Symposium itself is a document that proves that the ideas of Freud were being elaborated by Soviet academia way before the Symposium happened. This elaboration, however, was deeply grounded in experimental methodology and belonged to the discipline of physiology, rather than psychology. Although as we have discovered earlier in this book that the shift to the field of physiology was inevitable in the times of Pavlov's hegemony in science, further research went beyond reflexology and included complex theories like those of Anokhin and Bernstein. Another discipline where psychoanalysis found itself 'at home' in Soviet academia was philosophy, as many articles from the Symposium indicated, especially Lacanian psychoanalysis.

Importantly, materials of the Symposium served as an encyclopaedia of psychoanalytic texts, making them available for the wider audience. In times of censorship, it was a significant event, which in the tradition of the Freud Session in 1958 managed to keep the discussion around psychoanalysis ongoing.

## Freud and Soviet philosophers: *Voprosy Filosofii* and miscellaneous publications

In his book *The Unconscious in Soviet Tbilisi* [*Bessoznatel'noe v Sovetskom Tbilisi*] (2019) philosopher and psychoanalyst from Saint-Petersburg, Victor Mazin opens with the grandiosity of the Symposium 'he has not even participated in'. Mazin starts by stating no less than that the publication of Symposium materials in 1978[30] changed his life. Immediately after he notices that the 'myth of the disappearance' of psychoanalysis in the Soviet Union was repeated in the same way on both sides, in the West and in Russia (2019, p. 14).[31] He supports the view that psychoanalysis did not disappear after the 1930s, although its presence, "was dispersed in the discourse, in everyday life, in art" (p. 13).

Mazin first encountered Lacan in the paper written by Nataliia Avtonomova about Lacanian psychoanalysis (p. 26) that was published in one of the volumes, as well as writings by Serge Leclaire (1978) and Elisabeth Roudinesco (1978). In conversation with Mazin, Avtonomova remembers that she, in her turn, encountered Lacan years before the Symposium, when researching French structuralism as a doctoral student in philosophy. Through the National Library she was able to access Lacan's *Ecrits* (p. 86) for her research. It is amazing to imagine the presence of Lacan in someone's doctoral dissertation in the 1960s in a Soviet university!

Certainly Mazin was not the only person 'affected', although in the conclusion he shares memories of Avtonomova, who does not recall that the Symposium had any resonance in Moscow (Mazin, 2019, p. 134). Indeed, it was difficult to imagine that Soviet academia would pick up and openly start to discuss Freud after so many years of silence. Considering also that articles by Althusser, Anzieu, Clement, Green, Roundinesco were published in French, and the set of articles of American participants were in English, a lot of effort was required from the reader to obtain translations. However, Mazin asks (p. 147), does psychoanalysis really need official recognition? Even more, can psychoanalysis be translated into scientific language to be affirmed by academic institutions? This question brings us to the critique of the institutionalization of psychoanalysis, and the adverse effects of the collaboration of psychoanalysis with the state, the difficulties of standardization of training and elitism that arise from it, as well as the simplifications and distortions that psychoanalysis must undergo to fit into academia and study programs. As this book attempts to illustrate, the engagement with psychoanalysis can be productive, even if it takes place within academia or with the use of scientific methods. The work of Luria and Zeigarnik certainly can be a good example of it in clinical psychology and neuropsychology. Was the discussion around Freud in Soviet philosophy and psychology similarly productive?

As well as many others, Mazin was influenced by psychoanalytic thought that at times was not bound up with the clinical method or training institution. Instead, it was a knowledge that presented itself as a philosophy and worldview. Perhaps, it is not surprising that in the absence of psychoanalytic clinics, psychoanalytic theory was discussed by philosophers. Like others, however, philosophers such as Avtonomova could not openly engage with Freud except in a critical manner.

It is not surprising that the Journal *Voprosy Filosofii* [Issues of Philosophy] [32] hosted multiple discussions around the question of the unconscious or psychoanalysis or Freud (1956, 1957, 1958, 1959, 1960, 1961, 1962, 1963, 1966, 1967, 1968, 1969, 1970, 1971, 1972, 1973, 1975, 1976, 1977, 1978). Filipp Bassin was among regular authors; however, some other authors occasionally participated in the discussion around psychoanalysis and the question of the unconscious.

*Voprosy Filosofii* published a summary of Freud's session in 1959. The session dedicated to the philosophical questions of the physiology of higher nervous activity was also published in its pages in 1962 – both with the participation of Bassin. The resolution on the revival of psychology as a discipline appeared on its pages in 1963. In this period there was an open turn towards discussion of the problem of the unconscious, and it is notable that precisely in *Voprosy Filosofii* these events were discussed.

In the late 1960s and 1970s, Bassin continued to discuss psychophysiology, but he was also interested in psychological defence mechanisms, the question of ego strength and psychosomatic medicine (1967, 1968, 1969, 1970, 1971,

1975, 1978). For comparison, his articles in *Voprosy Psikhologii* [*Issues of Psychology*], another main journal, but in the psychology field, were not as frequent and were of a different kind. In 1958, they published Bassin's paper on the question of the unconscious – his speech at the Freud Session; in 1960 they published an exchange between Bassin and Musatti; in 1971 his review on the development of psychology; and in 1972 and 1973 articles about meaningful experiences and the development of meaning and signs.

*Voprosy Filosofii* even published two articles with some discussion of Lacanian ideas in 1973 (Avtonomova, 1973) and 1976 (Filippov, 1976), although predominantly dedicated to the structuralism movement in France. Without criticism, ideas of Lacanian psychoanalysis are presented in the light of his 'return to Freud', the mirror stage, narcissism, and the role of language in constructing the subject and the unconscious are given there. Overall, as a reader I got the impression that ideas of structuralism are not alien to Soviet ideology and there was no open critique of Lacan in these articles.

It is not surprising perhaps, that psychoanalysis was more accepted for discussion in the field of philosophy than in the field of psychology, a discipline, where remnants of the purges of the 1930s were still strong. However, there was also a critique of Freud from Soviet philosophers. As one of them, F.T. Mikhailov, remembers much later, in 2001,

> *Beyond the Threshold of Consciousness. A Critical Essay on Freudism*, published by Politizdat in 1961, was written by me in collaboration with G. I. Tsaregorodtsev (but separately by chapter, which is indicated on the back of the title). At that time, after a 30-year break, it became the first publication dedicated to Freud.[33] But even in the early sixties, things with psychoanalysis were not easy. Only a party publishing house could then risk such an ideologically dubious enterprise. And only 'in line with the fiercest struggle against bourgeois ideology'. Therefore, in *Beyond the Threshold of Consciousness* this struggle of ours is present and is perceived today as something ... beyond the threshold of decency. However, despite the fact that pretty soon I felt ashamed of the righteously angry invectives against the father of psychoanalysis, which took place even in my sections and chapters – and there are four of them out of five, every attentive reader will notice, accidentally getting acquainted with them and with what is said here in the same address that I did not become a follower of Freud.
>
> (Mikhailov, 2001, p. 640)

While reading this book, I concluded that Mikhailov did a lot to promote psychoanalysis. For a reader interested in knowing about Freud's theory, the book provided a comprehensive review of the history of the method, the theory of unconscious and ego, and the dissemination of psychoanalytic ideas in the West. For that, of course, a reader must be able, as Yurchak pointed out, to distance themself from the authoritarian discourse, to spare the internal space from the dictatorship of the official ideas. The reader must have been able to keep the split and to live in the double dimension, where "Freud was not right, and let's study him to know more how exactly". In that sense, the negation of Freud turned out to be a positive thing, as Freud himself argued in the work on negation. With the particle 'no', his ideas were preserved and available for the public.

\*

In this chapter it has become apparent that the theory of set formulated by Uznadze is not different from Freud's notion of the unconscious. Moreover, it is a productive elaboration of it, in many ways like the notion of unconscious phantasy as formulated by the Kleinian school. Through Bassin's efforts, the set became the Soviet alternative to the Freudian unconscious, however only on the level of vocabulary. On the level of understanding, this alternative Soviet unconscious did not exist. The difference in Soviet studies is present on the methodological level, as the unconscious was studied experimentally through observations. Reading through the materials of the Symposium in Tbilisi showed that the engagement with Freud's ideas was thoughtful and productive. Through the work of Uznadze and his school, the psychoanalytic idea of the unconscious received scientific support, and could be relevant in the ongoing discussion about the scientific status of psychoanalytic discoveries.

The return to archival materials around Bassin and reading of his main monographs, offers evidence of continuity in his interest in psychoanalytic theory, interrupted by ideological changes in science, rather than his personal change of mind. As with Luria, Bassin never 'abandoned' psychoanalysis and, when the opportunity was available, he continued to be engaged in research and the promotion of psychoanalytic ideas. He adopted the strategy of quasi-criticism and continued to bring psychoanalytic ideas to the discussion in disguise. Through his efforts, psychoanalytic theory never completely disappeared from the academic scene and many new names in psychoanalysis reached the Soviet reader through his publications and edited volumes. The Symposium on the Unconscious in Tbilisi, with its 4,000 participants, as well as personal stories about its impact, proves Bassin's effort to have been successful.

That again brings us to the idea of the trauma of the encounter of Soviet enthusiasts of psychoanalysis with state changes that occurred in the 1930s being displaced in current historiography to the dissatisfaction with psychoanalysis, rather than revealing the devastating consequences of purges and transformations in science. In my reading, I suggest putting back the affect of this traumatic encounter where it belongs – between an individual and the state. That interpretation allows us to free psychoanalytic theory from the negativity of the attitude and to see negation as the mechanism of a disguise technique that allowed for the conversation around psychoanalysis to keep going.

## Notes

1. GARF, f. P4737, o.2, d. 2143.
2. GARF, f.P-9506, o.16, d.213, p. 264.
3. Alexander Prangishvili was a Georgian psychologist, the head of the Institute of Psychology that was founded by Uznadze, the co-organizer from the Georgian side of the International Symposium on the Problem of Unconscious in Tbilisi in 1978. He was also an editor of three volumes of the materials, published prior to the symposium.
4. Irradiation is a term widely used in Soviet (and Russian) physiology and neurology to describe the spread of impulse to the areas that are physiologically outside of the zone where the impulse is applied. A good example of it is irradiation of pain (in English – radiation of pain).
5. Perhaps the experimental studies require a note for the psychoanalytic reader to situate it in their mind. I don't have an answer as to how Uznadze came to this experimental setting. In his writings the series of experiments usually appears without any preamble as to why and how he came to such experiment design. At times it appears as well as if the necessity for the experimental ground that was dictated by shifts in science was the reason for these experiments to be described, but the real value of his thinking is in the theoretical constructions around it.
6. Saying that, Uznadze also notes that there is no thought activity in animals, despite attempts by some bourgeois psychologists to suggest so. As he will later note, animals do not experience repetition, even though they are repeating the same acts, because in a true sense they are not experiencing them as the same. These views on thought and repetition being specifically human phenomena show that Uznadze separates the work of mind from the physiological activity of the brain and biological phenomena.
7. GARF, f.P-9506, o.16, d.213, p. 264.
8. GARF, f.P-9506, o.16, d.213, p. 264.
9. GARF, f.P-9506, o.16, d.213, p. 19.
10. Mikhail Livanov was a Soviet physiologist, a founder of the Soviet electroencephalography.
11. GARF, f.P-9506, o.16, d.213, p. 36 or GARF, f.P-9506, o.16, d.213, p. 74.
12. Semyon Sarkisov figure has been already discussed in previous chapters. He opened the Freud session in 1958, he was a member of the commission that discussed Luria's destiny, see footnote 18 in the Chapter 1.
13. Nikolai Grashchenkov Soviet neurologist, who played an important role in the career of Luria. See footnote 26 in Chapter 1 for more details.
14. GARF, f.P-9506, o.16, d.213, p. 32.
15. GARF, f.P-9506, o.16, d.213, p. 157.
16. GARF, f.P-9506, o.16, d.213, p. 160.
17. GARF, f.P-9506, o.16, d.213, p. 170.
18. Nikolai Bernstein was a Soviet psychophysiologist, who is famous for his study of motor activity, the unconscious mechanisms of movements. He was a son of the psychiatrist and psychotherapist Alexander Bernstein, who was in the first circles of enthusiasts of psychoanalysis in Russia before the Revolution.
19. GARF, f.P-9506, o.16, d.213, p. 178.
20. GARF, f.P-9506, o.16, d.213, pp. 19–25.
21. It is important to mention that according to the profile form Bassin knew German, English and French enough to read and to communicate in these languages (GARF, f.P-9506, o.16, d.213, p. 264). Hence, he was able to get access to updates in publications in the West, that would not be translated into Russian.

22 This article was also published in Italy, in *Revisita Pikoanalisi* in 1959 and initiated a 'dialogue' with Cesare Musatti, an Italian psychoanalyst, an editor of Italian edition of Freud's works. A full discussion with him was published in Bassin's monograph in 1968. This article most likely is a published version of Bassin's presentation in the Freud Session in 1958. As we know from preface to Alberto Angelini's book (1988), Musatti visited Soviet Union in 1967. Thus, by that time Bassin and Musatti had been in exchange for over 10 years.
23 From a personal exchange (November 2021). I'm thankful to Olga for her generous emails where she shared some memories about this time.
24 According to a librarian Linor Linza (personal exchange, November 2021), a special pass was given to scholars whose research thematically would allow them to read Freud. They could be doctors, philosophers, and psychologists.
25 But how would Bassin know about Lacan? Thanks to work of Natalia Avtonomova (Avtonomova, 1973) who was at that time already a Lacanian scholar. Her doctorate dissertation in 1973 was dedicated to the philosophical questions of structural analysis and had an extensive reflection on French structuralism. Her contribution to the further development of psychoanalysis, and of the Lacanian school after the fall of the Soviet Union was huge. She translated and edited *The Language of Psychoanalysis* by Laplanche and Pontalis (published in 1996) alongside Foucault's (1977) and Derrida's (2000) writings, no doubt circulated already in Soviet times.
26 A bit earlier in this section he also makes a remark about repression, saying that "although psychoanalysis does not offer a scientific explanation of the phenomena of repression, *it first makes it an indisputable fact of science*" (my italics) (p. 51). It is paradoxical that without a scientific explanation repression is here made an indisputable fact of science.
27 Sudakov and Kotov (1978).
28 Translation is taken from the original publication.
29 That explains to me in hindsight how Boris Veniaminovitch Iovlev, my former clinical supervisor and one of the eldest members at the Bekhterev Psychoneurological Institute in Saint-Petersburg, could know so much about Lacan. I remember when I just started as a doctorate candidate there with my research grounded in Lacanian theory, he said to me something like, "Finally I'll have someone to talk about Lacan with!".
30 As noted previously, the first three volumes of the symposium papers were published a year before the actual event, in 1978. An additional volume was published several years later, in 1985.
31 As his former student and a colleague, the way I think about the issue of disappearance of psychoanalysis and my curiosity on the topic were possibly formed in our conversations about the unconscious in Soviet times. This is something I had completely forgotten and only got reminded of when I read his book to prepare this chapter.
32 In this part I am relying on the archive of the issues of this journal for years 1958–1980, available in the Senate House Library, UCL SEESS library and the British Library.
33 As we know already, this was not exactly true, because by that time there were several articles dedicated to Freud, written by Bassin.

# Epilogue

In 2022, the *European Journal of Psychoanalysis* asked Alberto Angelini for his opinion on the current state of psychoanalysis in Russia. He replied:

> I am not aware of the developments of psychoanalysis in Russia in recent years; let's say in the third millennium. As a historian I worked essentially on the sources of the first half of the last century. Then some sketches on the situation until the eighties or a little more. From the few direct contacts I have had, I have come to the feeling that our Russian colleagues have, almost completely, neglected their glorious psychoanalytic past. It concerns both the last phase of the tsarist era, and the Soviet cultural world, until the mid-twenties of the twentieth century. It seems, but I hope to be proven wrong, that Russian psychoanalysts are currently flattening out on the contemporary features of the debate, especially as it unfolds in the US. This, probably, to try to conform to the "Western discourse" and to stay in tune with what is going on in the IPA. The greatest contribution of a Russian to the history of psychoanalysis in that country does not come from a psychoanalyst, but from a historian of literary training, Aleksandr Etkind, with the magnificent volume *Eros of the Impossible* (1993).

Indeed, being a discipline without its history, psychoanalysis in Russia after the fall of the Soviet Union had to start *as if* afresh and form a field consisting of translated knowledge and imported concepts. A valuable heritage got lost amid enthusiasm for incorporating the Western model. Was it a neglect of a deliberate kind, when anything Soviet could not be treated as valuable given years of atrocities and forced isolation? Was it a hunger for new knowledge? Was it a result of the IPA standardisation policies that would not accept any local knowledge as valid? Although my book did not intend originally to engage with answering these questions, some of my findings could shed light on the historical rupture that is so apparent to Angelini.

As I have argued in this book, the socio-political conditions from 1930 to 1980 allowed for psychoanalytic discussions to occur only in specific and constrained ways. A glorious period for psychoanalysis was followed by devastation and purges. Not surprisingly, then, after the decade of formal persecution, Luria has not mentioned Freud's name in his writings. As my research suggests, this didn't mean that his engagement with psychoanalytic ideas had been interrupted. Rather, it led to the emergence of something that we won't find in the ordinary history of psychoanalysis – a productive interdisciplinary collaboration. The shift toward physiology, both imposed and genuine, transformed the psychoanalytic vocabulary leading to an original elaboration on Freud's discoveries. Uznadze's theory of the set and later Luria's writing is an example of that. Also, through Luria and Vygotsky, Zeigarnik's pathopsychology, in my view, is a distant relative of psychoanalytic theory.

Years of real danger and persecution forced many individuals to live in the split, both in their private and professional lives. That led to paradoxes that I attempted to untangle – for example, the Freud Session in 1958 where speakers came together to reinstate their positions against psychoanalysis and the crowd that condemned Freud they were well too informed about events and developments in the field of psychoanalysis internationally. Or the paradoxes of Bassin's critique of Freud, that for readers with knowledge of Freud's writings sounded like an introduction to psychoanalysis in disguise. This was the time when pychoanalytic concepts were prohibited and at the same time circulated. Academics in 1960s discussed Lacan while, at the same time, it was claimed that psychoanalysis had been abandoned. That splitting was part of the survival strategies that had to be invented to protect people from persecutions of various kinds, depending on the decade we are looking at. Psychoanalysis, like sex in the USSR, had to be negated in order to be spoken about. This I believe to be an important discursive formation, that later not only puzzled historians of psychoanalysis in Soviet times but also led to the interruption between generations of academics and could explain why after the fall of the Soviet Union and the arrival of the new generation of psychoanalysts, Freud was easily seen as 'outdated'.

Overall, the history of psychoanalysis in Soviet Russia is as complex and paradoxical as the history of Soviet society itself. This book would not be possible without insights accumulated by social historians over the past few decades. To look back at this history full of trauma and devastation is not always easy – this could be one of the reasons for the start *as if* afresh that happened to psychoanalysis after the fall of the Soviet Union and the reluctance to include the names of early enthusiasts of psychoanalysis into the scope and instead to see them as 'simply trained for a new profession'.

This book also offers a contribution to the historiography of psychoanalysis that is interested in the interdisciplinary engagements of psychoanalysis, cultural influence or wild analysis. Ultimately, this is a history of psychoanalysis as a discipline of the unconscious that found ways to exist and adapt in diverse geographical and political contexts, independent of the narrative of great or mad men and situated on the outskirts of the major history of institutes of psychoanalysis. That is why this is the story of the vicissitudes of psychoanalysis.

*Vicissitudes* (noun, plural), according to the Cambridge Dictionary are "changes that happen at different times during the life or development of someone or something, especially those that result in conditions being worse". In psychoanalysis, 'vicissitudes' is a word that is normally attached to the notion of libido or drives, that relates to their changeability, to the capacity to alternate with the preservation of the initial impulse. I've chosen the word 'vicissitudes', and not 'destiny' or 'development', to think about changes that psychoanalysis went through in the particular period of Soviet history for that specific aspect of the meaning of the word. It is because the word 'destiny' would place figures of my research in the passive position, as if they had to agree with their fate and change, which I think was not at all the case. And if I used the word 'development', that would include the active position of my participants, but assume the replacement of old ideas with new, which I think was not at all the case either. So it is the word vicissitudes that is able to best reflect on the process of changing something while keeping it preserved.

Although Luria is sometimes called 'the father of the neuropsychology', Zeigarnik 'a pioneer of Soviet medical psychology', and Uznadze 'the great discoverer of the set', they all contributed to the productive elaboration of the role of the unconscious and language as regulators of the mental processes. More importantly, their work was at the core interdisciplinary and to me this is the most important discovery of the book: to preserve something, we don't have to keep it intact.

# References

Allen, A., and Ruti, M. (2019) *Critical Theory Between Klein and Lacan: A Dialogue*. London and New York, Bloomsbury Academic.

Angelini, A. (1988) *La psicoanalisi in Russia* [Psychoanalysis in Russia]. Napoli: Liguori.

Angelini, A. (2008) History of the Unconscious in Soviet Russia: From its Origins to the Fall of the Soviet Union. *International Journal of Psychoanalysis*, 89 (2): 369–388.

Arnold, O. (1999) Zvezdnyi Chas Filippa Veniaminovicha Bassina. *Priroda*, 10: pp. 98–105.

Avtonomova, N. (1973) Psikhoanaliticheskaia kontseptsiia Zhaka Lakana. *Voprosy Filosofii*, 11, s. 143.

Bassin, F. V. (1960) A Critical Analysis of Freudianism, *Soviet Review*, 1(5): 3–14.

Bassin, F. V. (1963) Soznanie i Bessoznatel'noie. *Filosofskie voprosy fiziologii vysshei nervnoi deiatel'nosti i psikhologii*. Moskva: Izdatel'stvo Akademii Nauk SSSR.

Bassin, F. V. (1968) *Problema Bessoznatel'nogo*. Moskva: Medicina.

Bassin, F. V. (1976) Predislovie. *Marksistskaia Kritika Psikhoanaliza*. Moskva: Progress.

Bassin, Yaroshevsky (ed.) (1991) *Sigmund Freid. Lektsii po Vvedeniiu v Psikhoanaliz*. Moskva: Nauka.

Bell, D. (2004) Reflections on the Death Drive: Commentary on 'The So-called Death Drive' by Jean Laplanche. *British Journal of Psychotherapy*, 20: 485–491. doi:10.1111/j.1752-0118.2004.tb00166.x.

Bell, D. L. (2015) The Death Drive: Phenomenological Perspectives in Contemporary Kleinian Theory. *International Journal of Psychoanalysis*, 96: 411–423. doi:10.1111/1745-8315.12212.

Bogdanchikov, S. A. (2002) Luria and Psychoanalysis. *Voprosy Psikhologii*, 4: 84–93.

Bogdanchikov, S. A. (2009) Sovremennye Otechestvennye Avtory o Nauchnykh Shkolakh v Sovetskoi Psikhologii v 1920–1930-h gg. (Opyt Detal'nogo Kriticheskogo Analiza). *Metodologija i Istorija Psihologii*, 4(2): C 7–31.

Bogdanchikov, S. A. (2018, September) *Thesis on the conference on the Soviet psychology*.

Bogdanchikov, S. A. (2020) *Stanovleniie Sovetskoi Psikhologii (1920–1930s)/ Uchebnoe posobie*. Moscow: Izdatel'stvo ASU.

Bondarenko, P. P., and Rabinovitch, M. X. (1959) The Scientific Session On the Questions of the Ideological Struggle Against Contemporary Freudism. *Problems of Philosophy*, 2: 164–170.

Brandenberger, D. (2005) Stalin as Symbol: A Case Study of the Personality Cult and Its Construction. In S. Davies, and J. Harris (eds), *Stalin: A New History* (pp. 249–270). Cambridge: Cambridge University Press.

Breuer, J., and Freud, S. (1893) *On The Psychical Mechanism of Hysterical Phenomena: Preliminary Communication from Studies on Hysteria.* The Standard Edition of the Complete Psychological Works of Sigmund Freud, Volume II (1893–1895): Studies on Hysteria, 1–17.

Brokman, A. (2018) Sterility and Suggestion: Minor Psychotherapy in the Soviet Union, 1956–1985. PhD thesis.

Brokman, A. (2018a) Sterility and Suggestion: Minor Psychotherapy in the Soviet Union, 1956–1985. *History of the Human Sciences*, 31(4): 83–106. doi:10.1177/0952695118773962.

Byford, A. (2020) *Science of the Child in Late Imperial and Early Soviet Russia.* Oxford University Press.

Buzin, V. N. (1995) Psychoanalysis in the Soviet Union: On the History of a Defeat. *Russian Social Science Review*, 36(6): 65–73. doi:10.2753/RSS1061–1428360665.

Calloway, P. (1992) *Russian/Soviet and Western Psychiatry: A Comparative Study.* Wiley

Cameron, L., and Forrester, J. (2017) *Freud in Cambridge.* United Kingdom: Cambridge University Press.

Chkhartishvili, S. N. (1978) K voprosu ob ontologicheskoi prirode bessoznatel☒nogo. *Bessoznatel'noe: Priroda, Funktsii, Metody Issledovaniia. Tom I. Razvitie Idei.* Tbilisi: Meznieriba.

Chukhrov, K. (2020) *Practicing the Good: Desire and Boredom in Soviet Socialism.* Minneapolis, MN: University of Minnesota Press.

Cole, M., and Levitin, K. (eds) (2006) *The Autobiography of Alexander Luria: A Dialogue with The Making of Mind.* Mahwah, NJ: Lawrence Erlbaum Associates.

Cote, M. (1998) *Russian Psychology in Transition.* Nova Science

Cordón, L. A. (2012) *Freud's World: An Encyclopedia of his Life and Times.* Greenwood.

Derrida, J. (1996) *Archive Fever: A Freudian Impression.* Chicago: University of Chicago Press.

Etchegoyen, R. H. (1999) *The Fundamentals of Psychoanalytic Technique.* London: Karnac.

Etkind, A. (1997) *Eros of the Impossible: The History of Psychoanalysis in Russia.* Boulder: Westview Press.

Feuer, L. (1987) Freud's Ideas in the Soviet Setting: A Meeting with Aleksandr Luriia. *Slavic Review*, 46(1): 106–112. doi:10.2307/2498623.

Figes, O. (2008) *The Whisperers: Private Life in Stalin's Russia.* United Kingdom: Penguin Books Limited.

Filippov, L. (1976) Strukturalizm i Freidizm. *Voprosy Filosofii*, 3: s.155.

Fink, B. (2017) *A Clinical Introduction to Freud: Techniques for Everyday Practice.* New York. W.W. Norton & Company.

Fitzpatrick, S. (1999) *Everyday Stalinism: Ordinary Life in Extraordinary Times: Soviet Russia in the 1930s.* New York: Oxford University Press.

Fitzpatrick, S. (2005) *Tear Off the Masks!: Identity and Imposture in Twentieth-century Russia.* United Kingdom: Princeton University Press.

Foucault, M. (1972) *The Archaeology of Knowledge.* London: Pantheon Books.

Fraser, J., and Yasnitsky, A. (2015) Deconstructing Vygotsky's Victimization Narrative: A Re-examination of the 'Stalinist Suppression' of Vygotskian Theory. *History of the Human Sciences*, 28(2): 128–153.

Freud, S. (1891) *On Aphasia. A Critical Study*. New York: International Universities Press.

Freud, S. (1895) *Project for a Scientific Psychology* (1950 [1895]). The Standard Edition of the Complete Psychological Works of Sigmund Freud 1: 281–391.

Freud, S. (1898) *The Psychical Mechanism of Forgetfulness*. The Standard Edition of the Complete Psychological Works of Sigmund Freud, Volume III (1893–1899): Early Psycho-Analytic Publications: 287–297.

Freud, S. (1900) *The Interpretation of Dreams*. The Standard Edition of the Complete Psychological Works of Sigmund Freud, Volume IV (1900): The Interpretation of Dreams (First Part): ix–627.

Freud, S. (1901) *The Psychopathology of Everyday Life: Forgetting, Slips of the Tongue, Bungled Actions, Superstitions and Errors* (1901) The Standard Edition of the Complete Psychological Works of Sigmund Freud, Volume VI (1901): The Psychopathology of Everyday Life: vii–296.

Freud, S. (1911) *Formulations on the Two Principles of Mental Functioning*. The Standard Edition of the Complete Psychological Works of Sigmund Freud, Volume XII (1911–1913): 213–226.

Freud, S. (1914b) *Remembering, Repeating and Working-Through (Further Recommendations on the Technique of Psycho-Analysis II)*. The Standard Edition of the Complete Psychological Works of Sigmund Freud, Volume XII (1911–1913): The Case of Schreber, Papers on Technique and Other Works: 145–156.

Freud, S. (1915) *The Unconscious*. The Standard Edition of the Complete Psychological Works of Sigmund Freud, Volume XIV (1914–1916): On the History of the Psycho-Analytic Movement, Papers on Metapsychology and Other Works: 159–215.

Freud, S. (1915b) *Instincts and their Vicissitudes*. The Standard Edition of the Complete Psychological Works of Sigmund Freud, Volume XIV (1914–1916): On the History of the Psycho-Analytic Movement, Papers on Metapsychology and Other Works: 109–140.

Freud, S. (1916) *Introductory Lectures on Psycho-Analysis*. The Standard Edition of the Complete Psychological Works of Sigmund Freud, Volume XV (1915–1916): Introductory Lectures on Psycho-analysis (Parts I and II): 1–240.

Freud, S. (1918) *From the History of an Infantile Neurosis*. The Standard Edition of the Complete Psychological Works of Sigmund Freud, Volume XVII: 1–124.

Freud, S. (1920) *Beyond the Pleasure Principle*. The Standard Edition of the Complete Psychological Works of Sigmund Freud, Volume XVIII (1920–1922): Beyond the Pleasure Principle, Group Psychology and Other Works: 1–64.

Freud, S. (1923) *The Ego and the Id*. The Standard Edition of the Complete Psychological Works of Sigmund Freud, Volume XIX (1923–1925): The Ego and the Id and Other Works: 1–66.

Freud, S. (1924) *The Loss of Reality in Neurosis and Psychosis*. The Standard Edition of the Complete Psychological Works of Sigmund Freud, Volume XIX (1923–1925): 181–188.

Freud, S. (1924a) *Neurosis and Psychosis*. The Standard Edition of the Complete Psychological Works of Sigmund Freud, Volume XIX: 147–154.

Freud, S. (1925) *A Note Upon the 'Mystic Writing-Pad'*. The Standard Edition of the Complete Psychological Works of Sigmund Freud, Volume XIX (1923–1925): The Ego and the Id and Other Works: 225–232.

Freud, S. (1925a) *Negation*. The Standard Edition of the Complete Psychological Works of Sigmund Freud, Volume XIX (1923–1925): The Ego and the Id and Other Works: 233–240.
Freud, S. (1926) *The Question of Lay Analysis*. The Standard Edition of the Complete Psychological Works of Sigmund Freud, Volume XX: 177–258.
Freud, S. (1927e) *Fetishism*. The Standard Edition of the Complete Psychological Works of Sigmund Freud, Volume XXI: 152–157.
Freud, S. (1933) *New Introductory Lectures On Psycho-Analysis*. The Standard Edition of the Complete Psychological Works of Sigmund Freud, Volume XXII: 1–182.
Freud, S., and Gay, P. (1995) *The Freud Reader*. London: Vintage.
Gilgen, A. R. (1997) *Soviet and American Psychology During World War II*. Praeger.
Ginzburg, C. (1989) *Clues, Myths, and the Historical Method*. Baltimore: Johns Hopkins University Press.
Goldman, W. Z. (1993) *Women, The State and Revolution. Soviet Family Policy and Social Life, 1917–1936*. Cambridge University Press.
Graham, L. (1967) *The Soviet Academy of Sciences and the Communist Party, 1927–1932*. Princeton, New Jersey.
Graham, L. (1988) *Science, Philosophy and Human Behaviour in the Soviet Union*. Columbia University Press.
Graham, L. (1993) *Science in Russia and the Soviet Union: A Short History*. New York: Cambridge University Press.
Hames, M. P. G. (2002) The Early Theoretical Development of Alexander Luria. PhD, University of London, UCL.
Healey, D. (2001) *Homosexual Desire in Revolutionary Russia: The Regulation of Sexual and Gender Dissent*. Chicago: University of Chicago Press.
Hill, P. (2002) *Using Lacanian Clinical Technique: an Introduction*. London: Press for the Habilitation of Psychoanalysis.
Homskaya, E. (2001) *Alexander Romanovich Luria: A Scientific Biography*. New York: Plenum Publishers.
Hook, D. (2017) *Six Moments in Lacan: Communication and Identification in Psychology and Psychoanalysis*. United States: Taylor & Francis.
Hristeva, G., and Bennett, P. W. (2018) Wilhelm Reich in Soviet Russia: Psychoanalysis, Marxism, and the Stalinist reaction. *International Forum of Psychoanalysis*, 27(1): 54–69, doi:10.1080/0803706X.2015.1125018.
Imedadze, I. (2009) Uznadze's Scientific Body of Work and Problems of General Psychology. *Journal of Russian & East European Psychology*, 47(3): 3–30, doi:10.2753/RPO1061-0405470301.
Jones P. (2006) *The Dilemmas of De-Stalinization. Negotiating Social and Political Change in the Khrushchev Era*. Routledge.
Joravksy, D. (1989) *Russian Psychology: A Critical History*. Blackwell.
Joseph, B. (1982) Addiction to Near Death. *International Journal of Psycho-Analysis*, 63: 449–456.
Jurinetz, V. (1924) Freidism i Marksism[Freudism and Marxism]. *Pod Znamenem Marksisma*, 8/9, 51–93.
Karpenko, L. A. (ed.) (2005) *Psikhologicheskii leksikon. Entsiklopedicheskii slovar' v shesti tomakh*. [Psychological lexicon. Encyclopaedic Dictionary in Six Volumes]. Moscow: PER SE.

Kadyrov, I. M. (2005) Analytical Space and Work in Russia: Some Remarks on Past and Present. *International Journal of Psychoanalysis*, 86(2): 467–482.

Kadyrov, I. M. (2013) Letter from Moscow. *International Journal of Psychoanalysis*, 94(2): 211–220.

Ketchuashvili, G. (2014) Dimitry Uznadze (1886–1950). *Transcultural Studies*, 10(3): 1–18.

Klein, M. (1946) Notes on Some Schizoid Mechanisms. *International Journal of Psycho-Analysis*, 27: 99–110.

Klein, M. (1959) Our Adult World and its Roots in Infancy. *Human Relations*, 12(4): 291–303. doi:10.1177/001872675901200401.

Kozulin, A. (1984) *Psychology in Utopia: Toward a Social History of Soviet Psychology*. Cambridge, MA: MIT Press.

Kozulin, A. (1989) Soviet Studies in the Psychodynamics of the Unconscious. *Studies in Soviet Thought*, 37(3): 237–245. Retrieved July 16, 2021, from www.jstor.org/stable/20100422.

Kozulin, A. (2005) The Concept of Activity in Soviet Psychology: Vygotsky, His Disciples and Critics. In H. Daniels (ed.), *An Introduction to Vygotsky*. London: Routledge.

Krementsov, N. (1996) *Stalinist Science*. Princeton University Press

Krylova, A. (2000) The Tenacious Liberal Subject in Soviet Studies. *Kritika: Explorations in Russian and Eurasian History*, 1(1): 119–146. doi:10.1353/kri.2008.0092.

Kuteliia, A. (1956) O printsipial'nykh pozitsiiakh teorii ustanovki D. N. Uznadze. *Voprosy Psikhologii*, 2: 28–37.

Lacan, J., Tomaselli, S., Forrester, J., and Miller, J. (1991) *The Seminar of Jacques Lacan. Book 2, The Ego in Freud's Theory and in the Technique of Psychoanalysis, (1954–1955)*. New York and London: Norton.

Lacan, J., Miller, J., and Grigg, R. (1993) *The Seminar of Jacques Lacan. Book 3. The Psychoses (1955–56)*. London: Routledge.

Ladaria, E. (2014) From Concept to Sign, and Back Again. The Soviet reception of psychoanalytic unconscious. Accessed online September 20, 2021 at: www.google.com/url?sa=t&rct=j&q=&esrc=s&source=web&cd=&ved=2ahUKEwjvx8KNjKz8AhUKQ8AKHfM0CJoQFnoECA0QAQ&url=https%3A%2F%2Fojs.iliauni.edu.ge%2Findex.php%2Fidentitystudies%2Farticle%2Fview%2F195%2F129&usg=AOvVaw3tj6MIu1A1zeKf4D8V4gU-.

Lagache, D. (1950) Définition et aspects de la psychanalyse. *Revue Francaise de Psychanalyse*, 14(3): 384–423.

Lagache, D. (1951) Quelques aspects du transfert. *Revue Francaise de Psychanalyse*, 15(3): 407–424.

Laplanche, J. (1976) *Life and Death in Psychoanalysis*. Baltimore, MD: Johns Hopkins University Press.

Laplanche, J., and Pontalis, J. B. (1973) *The Language of Psycho-Analysis*. London: Karnac.

Leibin, V. (1991) Repressirovannyi psikhoanaliz: Freid, Trotskii, Stalin [Repressed Psychoanalysis: Freud, Trotsky, Stalin]. *Rossiiskii psikhoanaliticheskii vestnik*, 1: 32–55.

Ledeneva, A. V. (1998) *Russia's Economy of Favours. Blat, Networking and Informal Exchange*. Cambridge University Press

Lepeshinskaya, O. (1945) *The Origin of Cells From Living Matter and the Part Played by Living Matter in the Organism*. Moscow: Academy of Science. Accessed online at: http://books.e-heritage.ru/book/10083898.

Luria, A. R. (1925) Psychoanalysis as a System of Monistic Psychology. In *The Selected Writings of A. R. Luria*. White Plains: M. E. Sharpe.

Luria, A. R. (1926) Die moderne mssische Physiologie und die Psychoanalyse [Modern Russian Physiology and Psychoanalysis]. *Internationale Zeitschrift für Psychoanalyse*, 12(1): 40–53.

Luria, A. R. (1959) Afaziia i Analiz Rechevykh Protsessov. *Voprosy Iazykoznaniia*, 2. Accessed online January 3, 2022 at: www.marxists.org/russkij/luria/1959/speech-process.pdf.

Luria, A. R. (1961) *The Role of Speech in the Regulation of Normal and Abnormal Behavior*. Liveright.

Luria, A. R. (1971) *Speech and The Development of Mental Processes of the Child. An Experimental Investigation*. London: Staples Press.

Luria, A. R. (1971) The Origin and Cerebral Organization of Man's Conscious Action. *XIX International Congress of Psychology: Proceedings; 27 July - 2 Aug. 1969* (pp. 37–52). The British Psychological Society.

Luria, A. R. (1977) Psychoanalysis as a System of Monistic Psychology. *Soviet Psychology*, 16(2): 7–45.

Luria, A. R. (1981) *Language and Cognition*. Wiley.

Luria, A. R. (2002) *Priroda Chelovecheskikh Konfliktov. Ob'ektivnoe Izuchenie Dezorganizatsii Povedeniia Cheloveka*. Moskva: Kogito-Tsentr.

Luria, E. (1994) *Moi Otets A. R. Luria* [My Father A. R. Luria]. Moscow: Gnozis.

MacLeod, C. M. (2020) Zeigarnik and von Restorff: The Memory Effects and the Stories Behind Them. *Memory and Cognition*, 48: 1073–1088. doi:10.3758/s13421-020-01033-5.

Marko, M. (2018) Life and Work of the Psychologist Bluma Zeigarnik (1901–1988). *Neurosciences and History*, 6(3): 116–124. Accessed online November 8, 2021 at: https://nah.sen.es/en/issues/lastest-issues/164-journals/volume-6/issue-3/412-life-and-work-of-the-psychologist-bluma-zeigarnik-1901-1988.

Mazin, V. (2018) Delo 'Bessoznatel'noe v sovetskom Tbilisi' [The case 'Unconscious in the Soviet Tbilisi]. *Lacanalia*, 28: 37–72. Accessed online August 15, 2020 at: www.lacan.ru/wp-content/uploads/2017/08/lcn028_not_a_toy.pdf.

Mazin, V. (2019) *Bessoznatel'noe v Sovetskom Tbilisi* [The Unconscious in Soviet Tbilisi]. VEIP.

Mdivani, K., Kechhuashvili, G., and Nadirashvili, S. (1956) K Discussii o Probleme Ustanovki. *Voprosy Psikhologii*, 6: 114–152.

Mikhailov, F. T. (2001) *Izbrannoe*. Moskva: Indrik.

Miller, M. A. (1998) *Freud and the Bolsheviks: Psychoanalysis in Imperial Russia and the Soviet Union*. New Haven: Yale University Press.

Nadirashvili, S. A. (1978) Zakonomernosti formirovaniia i deistviia ustanovok razlichnykh urovnei. In *Bessoznatel'noe: Priroda, Funktsii, Metody Issledovaniia. Tom I. Razvitie Idei*. Tbilisi: Meznieriba.

Naiman, E. (1997) *Sex in Public: The Incarnation of Early Soviet Ideology*. New Jersey: Princeton University Press.

Nikolaeva, V. V. (1987) *Vliianie Khronicheskoi Bolezni na Psikhiku: Psikhologicheskoe issledovanie*. [The impact of chronic illness on the psyche: Psychological research] Moscow: Izdatelstvo MGU.

Nikolaeva, V. V. (2003) B. V. Zeigarnik i patopsikhologiia [Zeigarnik and Pathopsychology]. *Psikhologicheskii Zhurnal*, 3: 13–21.

Nikolaeva, V. V. (2011) B. W. Zeigarnik and Pathopsychology. *Psychology in Russia: State of the Art*, 4: 176–193.

Nikolaeva, V. V., and Poliakov, I. F. (2016) Bliuma Vol'fovna Zeigarnik. Fenomen Zeigarnik (1900–1988). In *Vydaiushchiesia psikhologi Moskvy* (pp. 301–308). Moskovskiĭ Gosudarstvennyĭ Psikhologo-Pedagogicheskiĭ Universitet.

Nobus, D. (2000) *Jacques Lacan and the Freudian Practice of Psychoanalysis*. London: Routledge.

Omel'chenko, E. (2000) 'My body, my friend'? Provincial youth between the sexual and gender revolutions. In *Gender, State and Society in Soviet and Post-Soviet Russia* (p. 141). Routledge.

Orozco, J. A. N. (2021) Transitionality, Playing, Identification and Symbolization: Winnicott and Vygotsky. *Journal of Psychiatry Reform*, 10(9).

Ovcharenko, V. (1999) The History of Russian Psychoanalysis and the Problem of its Periodisation. *Journal of Analytical Psychology*, 44: 341–353.

Ovcharenko, V. (2000) *Rossiiskie Psikhoanalitiki* [Russian Psychoanalysts]. Accessed online September 11 2021 at: https://web.archive.org/web/20111021014904/http://www.psychosophia.ru/main.php?level=7&cid=5.

Ovcharenko, V. (ed.) (2006) Summa Psikhoanaliza. 19 Tomov [Encyclopaedia of Psychoanalysis, 19 Volumes]. Accessed online March 1, 2020 at: https://web.archive.org/web/20081231222410/http://www.psychosophia.ru/main.php?level=18.

Perrie, M. (2001) *The Cult of Ivan the Terrible in Stalin's Russia*. United Kingdom: Palgrave Macmillan.

Pisch, A. (2016) *The Personality Cult of Stalin in Soviet Posters, 1929–1953 /Archetypes, Inventions and Fabrications*. ANU Press. Accessed online May 21 2020 at: http://press-files.anu.edu.au/downloads/press/n2129/html/imprint.xhtml?referer=&page=2#.

Plamper, J. (2012) *The Stalin Cult: A Study in the Alchemy of Power*. New Haven, CT: Yale University Press.

Pollock, G. H. (1982) Psychoanalysis in Russia and the U.S.S.R.: 1908–1979. *The Annual of Psychoanalysis*, 10: 267–279.

Pollock E. (2006) *Stalin and the Soviet Science Wars*. Princeton University Press.

Prangishvili, A. (1977) Psikhologiia Soznanie I Bessoznatel'noe [Psychology consciousness and the unconscious]. *Literaturnaia gazeta*, 48: 13.

Prangishvili, A. S., Sherozia, A. E., and Bassin, F. V. (eds) (1978a) *Bessoznatel'noe: Priroda, Funktsii, Metody Issledovaniia. Tom I. Razvitie Idei*. Tbilisi: Meznieriba.

Prangishvili, A. S., Sherozia, A. E., and Bassin, F. V. (eds) (1978b) *Bessoznatel'noe: Priroda, Funktsii, Metody Issledovaniia. Tom II. Son. Klinika. Tvorchestvo*. Tbilisi: Meznieriba.

Prangishvili, A. S., Sherozia, A. E., and Bassin, F. V. (eds) (1978c) *Bessoznatel'noe: Priroda, Funktsii, Metody Issledovaniia.Tom III. Poznanie. Obshenie. Lichost'*. Tbilisi: Meznieriba.

Prangishvili, A. S., Sherozia, A. E., and Bassin, F. V. (eds) (1985) *Bessoznatel'noe: Priroda, Funktsii, Metody Issledovaniia. Tom IV. Rezul'taty Discussii*. Tbilisi: Meznieriba.

Proctor, H. (2016) 'A Country Beyond the Pleasure Principle': Alexander Luria, Death Drive and Dialectic in Soviet Russia, 1917–1930. *Psychoanalysis and History*, 18(2): 155–182.

Proctor, H. (2020) *Psychologies in Revolution Alexander Luria's 'Romantic Science' and Soviet Social History*. Palgrave.

Pushrakeva, T. N., and Romanov, Y. A. (2000) *To the History of Psychoanalysis in Ukraine.* How to Practice a Psychoanalytic Therapy in Periods of Social Instability, Kyiv, April 21 – May 1, 2000. Available at: www.academia.edu/61105355/К_истории_психоанализа_в_Украине.

Reich, R. (2018) *State of Madness: Psychiatry, Literature, and Dissent After Stalin.* United States: Cornell University Press.

Rotenberg, V. (2015) *Triumf bessoznatel'nogo: sbornik esse.* [The Triumph of the Unconscious]. Ridero: Kindle Edition.

Roudinesco, E. (1990) *Jaques Lacan & Co.: A History of Psychoanalysis in France, 1925–1985.* Chicago: University of Chicago Press.

Rozhdestvenskii, D. (2009) *Psikhoanaliz v rossiiskoi kul'ture: uchebno-metodicheskoe posobie* [Psychoanalysis in Russian Culture: A Handbook]. VEIP.

Rustin, M. (2016) The Totalitarian Unconscious. In M. Ffytche, and D. Pick (eds), *Psychoanalysis in the Age of Totalitarianism.* Abingdon: Routledge

Salecl, R. (2011) *The Tyranny of Choice.* Profile Books

Santiago-Delefosse, M. J., and Delefosse, J.-M. O. (2002) Spielrein, Piaget and Vygotsky. *Theory & Psychology*, 12(6): 723–747.

Savelli, M., and Marks, S. (eds) (2015) *Psychiatry in Communist Europe.* Palgrave

Schur, M. (1966) *The Id and the Regulatory Principles of Mental Functioning.* New York: International Universities Press, Inc.

Sherozia, A. (1978) Psikhoanaliz i teoriia neosoznavaemoĭ psikhologicheskoĭ ustanovki: itogi i perspektivy. *Bessoznatel'noe: Priroda, Funktsii, Metody Issledovaniia. Tom I. Razvitie Idei.* Tbilisi: Meznieriba.

Shevrin, H. (1978) Neuropsychological Correlates of Psychodynamic Unconscious Processes. *Bessoznatel'noe: Priroda, Funktsii, Metody Issledovaniia. Tom I. Razvitie Idei.* Tbilisi: Meznieriba.

Shoshin, P. B. (1985) Puti kontseptualizatsii bessoznatel'nogo. Bessoznatel'noe: Priroda, Funktsii, Metody Issledovaniia. *Tom IV. Rezul'taty Discussii.* Tbilisi: Meznieriba.

Shoshin, P. B. (1992) Pamiati F. V. Bassina [In memory of F. V. Bassin]. *Konsul'tativnaia psikhologiia i psikhoterapiia. Tom 1. # 1.*

Shuster, A. (2016) One or Many Antisexes? Introduction to Andrei Platonov's "The Anti-Sexus". *Stasis*, 4(1): 20–35.

Silbermann, I. (1961) Synthesis and Fragmentation. *The Psychoanalytic Study of the Child*, 16: 90–117.

Sirotkina, I., and Smith, R. (2016) *History of Psychology in Russia: Short Review with the Authors' Emphasis* [Electronic resource]: Working paper WP6/2016/01.

Sokolova, E. T. (1976) *Motivatsiia i Vospriiatie v Norme i Patologii* [Motivation and Perception in Norm and Pathology]. Moskva: Izdatel'stvo Moskovskogo Universiteta.

Solms, M. (2000) Freud, Luria and the Clinical Method. *Psychoanalysis and History*, 2 (1): 76–109.

Spielrein, S. (1921) Russische Literatur. Bericht über die Fortschritte der Psychoanalyse in den Jahren 1914–1919 [Russian Literature on psychoanalysis]. *Beihefte der IZP*, 3: 356–365.

Spitz, R. A. (1964) The Derailment of Dialogue – Stimulus Overload, Action Cycles, and the Completion Gradient. *Journal of the American Psychoanalytic Association*, 12: 752–775.

Sudakov, K. V., and Kotov, A. V. (1978) Neuropsychological mechanisms of conscious and unconscious manifestations of biological motivations. *Bessoznatel'noe: Priroda, Funktsii, Metody Issledovaniia. Tom I. Razvitie Idei.* Tbilisi: Meznieriba.

Suny, R. G. (2011) *The Soviet Experiment. Russia, the USSR, and the Successor States.* Oxford University Press.

Szasz, T. S. (1958) The Role of the Counterphobic Mechanism in Addiction. *Journal of the American Psychoanalytic Association*, 6: 309–325.

Tögel, C. (2006) *Psychoanalysis and Communism: Freud in the early Soviet Union – Hope and Disappointment.* Freud-Symposium Budapest, June 22, 2006. Accessed online at: www.freud-biographik.de/publikationen/.

Uznadze, D. N. (1966) *The Psychology of Set.* New York: Consultants Bureau.

Voslensky, M. (1984) *Nomenklatura: The Soviet Ruling Class.* Garden City, NY: Doubleday.

Vyrgioti, M. (2021) Freud and the Cannibal: Vignettes from Psychoanalysis' Colonial History. In S. Bar-Haim, E. S. Coles, and H. Tyson (eds), *Wild Analysis: From the Couch to Cultural and Political Life* (pp. 67–81). Routledge.

Waterlow, J. (2018) *It's only a Joke, Comrade! Humour, Trust and Everyday Life under Stalin (1928–1941).* CreateSpace Independent Publishing Platform.

Weiskopf, M. (2001) *Pisatel' Stalin.* Moskva: Novoe Literaturnoe Obozrenie.

Yakushko, O. (2021) The Exclusion of Psychoanalysis in Academic and Organized U. S. Psychology: On Voodooism, Witch-Hunts, and the Legion of Followers, *Psychoanalytic Inquiry*, 41(8): 638–653. doi:10.1080/07351690.2021.1983405.

Yaroshevsky, M. G. (1988) V shkole Kurta Levina (Iz besed s B. V. Zejgarnik) [In the school of Kurt Lewin. From the conversation with Bluma Zeigarnik]. *Voprosy Psikhologii*, 3: 172.

Yasnitsky, A. (2009) Vygotsky Circle during the decade of 1931–1941: Toward an integrative science of mind, brain, and education. University of Toronto: ProQuest Dissertations Publishing.

Yasnitsky, A. (2012a) Izoljacionizm sovetskoj psihologii? Neformal'nye lichnye svjazi uchenyh, mezhdunarodnye posredniki i 'import' psihologii [Isolationism of Soviet psychology? Informal personal networks of scientists, international brokers, and import of psychology]. *Voprosy Psikhologii*, 1: 110–112.

Yasnitsky, A. (2012b) K istorii kul'turno-istoricheskoj geshtal'tpsihologii: Vygotskij, Lurija, Koffka, Levin i dr. [To the question of cultural-historical gestalt psychology: Vygotsky, Luria, Koffka, Lewin and others]. *Psihologicheskij zhurnal Mezhdunarodnogo universiteta prirody, obshhestva i cheloveka*, 1: 60–97.

Yasnitsky, A (2015) *Distsiplinarnoe stanovlenie russkoi psikhologii pervoi poloviny XX veka // Nauki o cheloveke: istoriia distsiplin* [The disciplinary formation of the Russian psychology of the first half of the 20th century // Sciences of man: the history of disciplines] Publishing House of NIU HSE.

Yasnitsky, A., and van der Veer, R. (eds) (2015) *Revisionist Revolution in Vygotsky Studies: The State of the Art.* United Kingdom: Taylor & Francis.

Yasnitsky, A. (ed.) (2019) *Questioning Vygotsky's Legacy: Scientific Psychology Or Heroic Cult.* United Kingdom: Taylor & Francis.

Yaroshevsky M. G. (1988) V shkole Kurta Levina (Iz besed s B. V. Zejgarnik) [In the school of Kurt Lewin. From the conversation with Bluma Zeigarnik]. *Voprosy Psikhologii*, 3: 172.

Yurchak, A. (2005) *Everything Was Forever, Until It Was No More: The Last Soviet Generation*. United States: Princeton University Press.

Zajicek, B. (2009) Scientific Psychiatry in Stalin's Soviet Union: the Politics of Modern Medicine and the Struggle to Define 'Pavlovian' Psychiatry, 1939–1953. PhD thesis, University of Chicago

Zajicek, B. (2014) Soviet Madness. *Ab Imperio*, 4: 167–194.

Zajicek, B. (2018) Soviet psychiatry and the origins of the sluggish schizophrenia concept, 1912–1936. *History of the Human Sciences*, 2: 88–105.

Zalkind, A. B. (1924) *The Twelve Sexual Commandments of the Revolutionary Proletariat*. Moscow: Ya. M. Sverdlov Communist University.

Zavershneva, E., and van der Veer, R. (eds) (2018) *Vygotsky's Notebooks. A Selection*. Springer.

Zavershneva, E. (2019) Psikhoz, iazyk i svoboda povedeniia. *Voprosy Psikhologii*, 1: 101–113.

Zeigarnik, A. V. (2001) Bliuma Vol'fovna Zeigarnik (popytka vosproizvedeniia zhiznennogo puti) [Bluma Zeigarnik. An attempt to recreate the life path]. *Konsul'tativnaja psikhologiia i psikhoterapiia*, 4: 182–193.

Zeiigarnikovskie chteniia [Zeigarnik's readings] (2020) *Conference materials*. Accessed online November 21, 2021 at: http://confzejgarnik.tilda.ws.

Zeigarnik, B. V. (1934) *K probleme ponimanija perenosnogo smysla slov ili predlozhenija pri patologicheskih izmenenijah myshlenija*. Moskva: Novoe v Uchenii ob Apraksii, Agnozii i Afazii.

Zeigarnik, B. V. (1958) *Narushenie myshleniia u psikhicheski bol'nykh* [Thought disorder in the mentally ill]. Moscow.

Zeigarnik, B. V. (1962) *Patologiya myshleniia* [Pathology of Thinking]. Moscow: Izdatelstvo Moskovskogo Universiteta.

Zeigarnik, B. V. (1965) *The Pathology of Thinking*. New York: Consultants Bureau.

Zeigarnik, B. V. (1969) *Vvedenie v patopsikhologiiu* [Introduction to Pathopsychology] Moscow: Izdatelstvo Moskovskogo Universiteta.

Zeigarnik, B. V. (1972) *Experimental Abnormal Psychology*. Monographs in Psychology. Boston, MA: Springer.

Zeigarnik, B. V. (1973) *Osnovy patopsikhologii* [Foundations of Psychopathology]. Moscow: Izdatelstvo Moskovskogo Universiteta.

Zeigarnik, B. V., Bakanova S. V., Nikolaeva V. V., and Sheftelevich O. S. (1978) The Attitude to one's Illness as a Condition for the Emergence of Conscious and Unconscious Motives of Activity. *Bessoznatel'noe* [The Unconscious]. Tbilisi: Metsniereba.

Zeigarnik, B. V. (1981) *Teoriia lichnosti Kurta Levina* [The Theory of Personality of K. Lewin]. Moscow: Izdatelstvo Moskovskogo Universiteta.

Zeigarnik, B. V. (1982) *Teorii lichnosti v zarubezhnoi psikhologii* [Theories of personality in foreign psychology]. Moscow: Izdatelstvo Moskovskogo Universiteta.

Zeigarnik, B. V. (1986) *Patopsikhologiia* [Pathopsychology]. Moscow: Izdatelstvo Moskovskogo Universiteta.

Zeigarnik, B. V., Bodalev, A. A., and Leont'ev, D. A. (1987) Problema Bessoznatel'nogo: dvizhenie k dialogu [The problem of the unconscious: Move to a dialogue]. *Voprosy Psikhologii*, 4: 163–165.

Zeigarnik, B. V. (2001) *Zapominanie zakonchennyh I nezakonchennyh deistvii* [Memorising finished and unfinished actions]. Moscow: Smysl.

Zolotova, N. V. (2007) Psikhologicheskie vozzreniia B. V. Zejgarnik [Psychological views of Zeigarnik]. PhD dissertation.

Zolotova, N. V. (2007a) Nauchnoe nasledie i zhiznennyii put' B. V. Zejgarnik [B. W. Zeigarnik's scientific heritage and life]. *Methodology and History of Psychology*, 2(2): 135–146.

# Index

abnormal psychology 100
abortion 61
Abraham, Karl 25, 30–31, 66, 144
Academy of Medicine 45, 51
Academy of Pedagogical Sciences 45
Academy of Sciences 41, 45
alcohol addiction 103
Alexander, Franz 54
Alexandrov, Grigori 71
All-Russian Psychoanalytic Society 84
All-Union Conference on Philosophical Issues in the Physiology of Higher Nervous Activity and Psychology (1962) 1, 45, 92, 147
Althusser, Louis 154, 159
Angelini, Alberto 2, 5–6, 27, 31, 34–36, 137, 164
Anokhin, Pyotr K. 4, 6, 54, 73–75, 118, 140, 142, 148, 158
anorexia nervosa 103
anti-Semitic campaign (1948–1953) 91–92, 117
Anzieu, Didier 141, 154, 159
aphasia 4, 11, 32, 84, 90–91, 96, 99, 117, 119, 125
archives 13–15
Arnold, Olga 144
Asatiani, Mikheil 25, 30
associative experiment 97
authoritarianism 17, 52, 55, 145, 161
authoritative discourse 18–20, 37, 64, 67
Averbukh, V.A. 26
Avtonomova, Nataliia 154, 158–159

Bakhtin, Mikhail 18, 25
Barnett, B. 156
Bassin, Filipp 3, 6–10, 13, 17, 25, 46, 49, 52–53, 57, 74–75, 85, 92–93, 107, 129–130, 132–133, 139–151, 154–157, 159–161, 165; birthplace of 7; *Problem of the Unconscious, The* (1968) 141, 143; return to Freud 142–143; unconscious 143–145
Baulieu, Emile 43
behaviourism 132
Bekhterev, V. M. 100
Bekhterev Psychoneurological Institute 31, 100
Bely, Andrey 25
Bennett, P. W. 66
Bernstein, Alexander 4, 25, 30, 158
Bernstein, Nikolai 118, 140, 142
Bertolucci, Bernardo 68
*Beyond the Pleasure Principle* (Freud, 1920) 29, 66–67
Bion, Wilfred 10, 56
Birenbaum, Gita 83
*blat* 20, 46
Bogdanchikov, Sergei 23–24, 118
brain damage 11, 52, 90–91, 99, 110–111, 119–120, 139
Brezhnev, Leonid 37, 39–40, 99
British Psychological Society 90
Brokman, Alexandra 76
Bruno, Pierre 149
Bukharin, Nikolai 69
Byford, Andy 55
Bzhalava, I. T. 133

Calloway, P. 50
Cameron, Laura 56
capitalism 12, 43
castration 48
censorship 5, 16, 23, 41, 48, 50–53, 65, 83, 85, 125, 158

Charcot, Jean-Martin 54
Chertok, Leon 154
Chukhrov, Keti 29
classification 88, 99
Clément, Catherine 149
Clement, Catrin 154, 159
clinical development 30–34
Cole, Michael 88
Collectivization 41
colonialism 12, 54–55
comradeship 38
criminal behaviour 88–89
crosshatching 20

Dali, Salvador 68
death drive 10, 28–29, 53
defectology 28, 110
denial 48
Derrida, Jacques 18, 142
de-Stalinization 2, 17, 39, 45
Diagnostic and Statistical Manual 101
disavowal 48
*Disturbances of Thinking of Psychiatric Patients* (Zeigarnik, 1958) 96
divorce 61–62
Doctor's Plot 91–92, 117
Dostoevsky, Fyodor 31–33, 68, 70
doublethink 48
dreams 5, 16, 31, 54, 69–70, 133, 137
*Drives and their Vicissitudes* (Freud, 1915) 56
dynamic stereotype 148

ego 29, 48, 53, 123, 125, 150, 159
*Ego and the Id, The* (Freud, 1923) 67, 123
Eisenstein, Sergei 25
electroencephalography 52, 139–140
electroshock 77
encyclopaedias 35–36
Engels, Friedrich 20, 67
Era of Stagnation 39
Ermakov, Ivan 25, 27, 31, 33, 66–67
Etkind, Alexander 2, 26–27, 32, 34, 50, 84, 164
*European Journal of Psychoanalysis* 164
evidential/conjectural paradigm 15–17
*Experimental Abnormal Psychology* (Zeigarnik, 1972) 93

family codes 61–2
Fedotov, Dmitry 54

Fellini, Federico 68
Ferenczi, Sandor 25, 31, 144
fetishism 48, 82
Fifth Five-Year Plan 41
Figes, O. 14
Filippov, L. 154
First Five-Year Plan 37–38
Fitzpatrick, S. 38, 44, 52
Five-Year Plans 62; First 37–38; Second 69, 77; Third 40; Fifth 41
foreclosure 48
Forrester, John 56
Foucault, Michel 14
*Foundations of Psychopathology* (Zeigarnik, 1973) 92
Freud, Rosa 71
Freud, Sigmund 9–10, 30–36, 43–44, 48–56, 81, 84–85, 87–89, 91, 98–99, 103–104, 129–130, 135–138, 141–161, 165; *On Aphasia* (1891) 122–123; becoming 'not legitimate' 65–8; *Beyond the Pleasure Principle* (1920) 29, 66–67; *On Children's Neuroses* (1925) 67; *Drives and their Vicissitudes* (1915) 56; *Ego and the Id, The* (1923) 67, 123; *Interpretation of Dreams* (1900) 5, 16, 25, 123; Introductory Lectures on Psychoanalysis 65–66; Luria on 107–109, 112–116, 118–125; *Project for a Scientific Psychology, The* (1895) 142; *Psychopathology of Everyday Life, The* (1901) 72; in the public discourse 60–77; *Question of Lay Analysis* (1926) 32; *Remembering, Repeating and Working Through* (1914) 144; and Soviet philosophers 158–161; *Three Essays on the Theory of Sexuality* (1924) 155; *Totem and Taboo* (1913) 69; *Unconscious, The* (1915) 87; Zeigarnik on 93–95, 104, *see also* Freudism
Freud Session (1958) 1–3, 5–6, 8, 10, 20, 36, 43, 45, 52, 54–55, 68, 73, 132, 150, 158, 160, 165
Freudian slips *see* slips of the tongue
Freudism 1–6, 26, 35–36, 45, 51–52, 55; becoming 'not legitimate' 65–69; dreams 5, 16, 31, 54, 69–70, 133, 137; fetishism 48, 82; Freud Session *see* Freud Session (1958); negation 43–46; Oedipus complex 10, 55, 67, 150; in the public discourse 60–77; repression

36,48; sexuality 9, 12, 31, 33, 54, 60–63, 67; slips of the tongue 16, 31, 63, 94, 102, 147, 151, 155
Freudomarxism 28

Gagarin, Alexei 115–116
Gedevanishvili, D. 131–132
Gestalt psychology 24, 67, 83, 86, 132
Gilgen, A. R. 28
Ginzburg, Carlo 16
Graham, Loren 27, 41, 50–51
Grashchenkov, N. I. 54, 140
Great Break 41
Great Patriotic War 23, 40
Green, Andre 141, 154, 159
Grozny, Ivan 41

Hartmann, Heinz 53
higher nervous activity 29, 42, 45, 73, 92, 143, 146–147, 159
Hitchcock, Alfred 68
homosexuality 61–62
Homskaya, E. 110, 118
Hristeva, G. 66
humour 17, 20, 31, 39–40, 47–48, 84, 123, 136
Hungarian Psychoanalytic Society 25
hypochondria 103
hysteria 100, 138

idealization in science 41–42
Imedadze, I. 129
internal emigration 40
International Congress of Psychology 90
International Symposium on the Unconscious (1979) 10, 63, 74, 93, 103, 129, 138–139, 141–142, 150–158, 161
*Internationale Zeitschrift für Psychoanalyse* 109
*Interpretation of Dreams* (Freud, 1900) 5, 16, 25, 123
*Introduction to Pathopsychology* (Zeigarnik, 1969) 82, 92–94, 119
IPA 31, 74, 164
*Izvestiia* 65–66, 68–70

Jacobson, Roman 156
jokes *see* humour
Jones, Ernest 25, 31, 66
Jones, P. 39

Jung, Carl 25, 30–31, 54, 66, 88, 97, 104, 109
Jurinetz, V. 66

Kakabadze, V. L. 133
Kannabikh, Yuri 25, 30, 35
Karvasarskii, Boris 74
Kazan Psychoanalytic Group 84, 107
Kerbikov, Oleg 53
Ketchuashvili, G. 129
Khrushchev, Nikita 17, 37, 39–40, 45, 49
Klein, Melanie 10–11, 25, 31, 41, 56, 133, 144, 152–153, 157, 161
Kolbanovskii, Victor 112, 116
*kommunalka* 38
Kornilov, Konstantin 43, 66–67, 111–116
Korsakov, S. S. 100
*Korsakov Journal* 100
Kozulin, Alex 2, 20, 27–28, 44, 129, 141
Krementsov, N. 20, 27, 37, 44, 51–52
Kris, Ernst 53
*Krokodil* 65, 68–70
Krylova, Anna 20–21, 85
*kulturnost* 37
Kuteliia, A. A. 131–132

Lacan, Jacques 10, 56, 81, 142, 150, 153, 155–156, 158, 160
Ladaria, E. 129
language 29, 36–43, 46, 64, 86–88, 90–91, 97–98, 103–104, 108, 118–125, 160
*Language and Cognition* (Luria, 1981) 123
Laplanche, Jean 10, 48
Lebedinskii, M. S. 51
Leclaire, Serge 156, 158
Ledeneva, A. V. 20, 44, 46–47
Lenin, Vladimir 20, 25–26, 28, 67, 92, 141
Leninism 18, 115
Leontiev, D. A. 91, 152
Lepeshinskaya, O. 41–42
Lewin, Kurt 83–85, 93–94, 105
libido 10, 62–63, 166
*Literaturnaia gazeta* 65, 67–68, 70–75, 131
Livanov, M. N. 139
lobotomy 77
Loewenstein, Rudolph 53
London University 90

Luria, Alexander 3–4, 6–9, 11–13, 16–17, 24, 26–29, 32, 35, 38, 46, 49, 51–52, 57, 66–67, 77, 81–85, 88–93, 97, 105, 107–125, 141–142, 149, 159, 161, 165–166; associative experiment 97; and the brain 110–118; co-operation with Zeigarnik 88–91; on Freud 107–109, 112–116, 118–125; history of 84–85, 88–89, 108–116; on language 108, 118–125; *Language and Cognition* (1981) 123; method of pictograms 98; *Nature of Human Conflicts, The* (1932) 88–89, 109–110, 112, 114; neuropsychology 9, 32, 43, 107–108, 110, 118, 125, 159, 166; persecution of 51; *Restoration of Function after Brain Injury* (1963) 91; *Role of Speech in the Regulation of Normal and Abnormal Behavior, The* (1961) 121; on schizophrenia 81, 100; search for a new science 108–110; on sexuality 60; *Speech and The Development of Mental Processes of the Child* (1956) 120; *Traumatic Aphasia* (1970) 91
Luria, E. 110–111, 117
Lysenko, Trofim 41–42

MacLeod, C. M. 85
Main, Tomas F. 154
Marko, M. 85
Markov, Michail 70
Marx, Karl 20, 28–29, 67, 92, 141
Marxism 2–3, 18, 27–30, 34–35, 43, 49, 54, 65–66, 113, 115, 147, 149–150
Marx-Lenin University 115
Mazin, Victor 158–159
melancholia 10
Meyer, Adolph 110
Meynert, Theodor 54
Miasishchev, V. N. 6, 31, 54
Michurin, Ivan 42
Mikhailov, F. T. 160
Mikhailov, Vladimir 74
Miller, Martin 2, 5–6, 27, 34, 50
mirror stage 160
Moscow State University 91–92, 94, 104
Musatti, Cesare 107, 144, 154, 160

Naiman, Eric 63
narcissism 69, 136, 160
*Nature of Human Conflicts, The* (Luria, 1932) 88–89, 109–110, 112, 114

*Nedelia* 65, 68
negated psychoanalysis 34–46
negation 43–46, 60, 151
Neo-Freudian movement 53
neo-Freudians 53, 93, 104, 109
neuropsychology 9, 11, 32, 43, 56, 107–108, 110, 118, 125, 155, 159, 166
Nevsky, Alexander 41
Nietzsche, Friedrich 54
Nikolaeva, V. V. 91, 103
Nixon, Richard 39
*novyi byt* 37

objectivization 137–138
October Revolution 27, 33, 35, 60–62, 85
Oedipus complex 10, 55, 67, 150
*Ogonek* 65, 68–69, 71
*On Aphasia* (Freud, 1891) 122–123
*On Children's Neuroses* (Freud, 1925) 67
Orwell, George 48
Osipov, Nikolay 25, 27, 30–31
Ovcharenko, Victor 22–24, 31

pansexuality 63
*Pathology of Thinking* (Zeigarnik, 1962) 96–97
pathopsychological experiment (Zeigarnik) 81–82, 88, 94, 97, 101, 105, 119
pathopsychology 9, 11, 28, 45, 81–82, 86, 88, 91–96, 99–105, 119, 125, 165
Pavlov, Ivan 18–19, 24, 42–43, 45, 53, 73, 75, 92, 116, 130, 132, 138, 140, 144, 148, 154–155, 158, *see also* Pavlovianism
Pavlov Session (1950–1951) 1–2, 12, 33, 37, 42, 44–45, 73, 117, 142
Pavlovianism 1–2, 4, 6, 19, 43, 54, 73, 95, 100, 131; Pavlov Session *see* Pavlov Session (1950–1951)
pedology 17, 28, 55, 111–112
*Personality and Pathology of Activity* (Zeigarnik, 1971) 92
Pevzner, M.S. 26
phantasy 99, 103, 133, 152, 157, 161
physiology 1–2, 6, 8–13, 16, 18, 29–30, 32, 37, 42–43, 45, 53–54, 56, 66, 73, 85, 92, 95, 107–110, 115, 118, 125, 131, 138, 142, 155, 158–159, 165
Piaget, Jean 24, 84
pictograms 98
Platonov, Andrei 62
*Pod Znamenem Marxisma* 66

Pollock, E. 20, 42
Popov, Evgeny 53, 62
poverty 38
Prangishvili, Alexander 74, 132, 138, 155
*Pravda* 18, 62–63, 65–70, 73, 146
*Problem of the Unconscious, The* (Bassin, 1968) 141, 143
Proctor, Hanna 3, 12, 29, 89, 110
*Project for a Scientific Psychology, The* (Freud, 1895) 142
*Psikhoterapiia* 30
Psychoanalytic Institute 25–26, 75
*Psychoanalytic Review* 110
psychocorrection 102
psychohygiene 28, 95
Psychological and Psychoanalytic Library 25, 31
*Psychology of Set, The* (Uznadze, 1966) 132–133
psychomarxism 150
psychopathology 32, 102, 137
*Psychopathology of Everyday Life, The* (Freud, 1901) 72
psychosomatic medicine 53, 74, 140, 143, 145, 155, 159
psychotechnics 28
purges 12, 14, 21, 26, 33, 38, 40–41, 84, 113, 141, 160–161, 165
Pushrakeva, T. N. 25

*Question of Lay Analysis* (Freud, 1926) 32

racism 114
reactology 28
reality principle 97, 103, 133
reflexology 4, 18, 28–29, 66, 73, 132, 142, 158
Reich, R. 39
Reider, Norman 54
*Remembering, Repeating and Working Through* (Freud, 1914) 144
repression 36, 48
*Restoration of Function after Brain Injury* (Luria, 1963) 91
*Role of Speech in the Regulation of Normal and Abnormal Behavior, The* (Luria, 1961) 121
Rollins, Nancy 74
Romanov, Y. A. 25
Rorschach test 86
Rosental, Tatiana 25, 31

Roudinesco, Elisabeth 27, 33, 43, 158–159
Rozanov, Vasily 25
Rozhdestvenskii, Dmitrii 2–3, 27, 30–33, 50
Rubinstein, Sergei 117
Rubinstein, Susanna 83
Russian Psychoanalytic Society 25, 31–32, 65–67, 70, 84, 89, 107, 109
Russification 7–8, 27
Russocentrism 42–43
Rustin, Michael 43–44

Sacks, Oliver 110
Salome, Lou-Andreas 25
Sarkisov, Semyon 52–53, 140
schizophrenia 4, 9, 13, 48, 81–82, 87, 90, 92, 94–104, 138–140
Schmidt, Otto 25, 27, 31
Schmidt, Vera 25–27
Schopenhauer, Arthur 54
Scientific Meeting on the Problem of the Ideological Struggle Against Contemporary Freudism *see* Freud Session (1958)
Sechenov, Ivan 24, 97
Second Five-Year Plan 69, 77
secret speech (Khrushchev) 17, 45, 49
self-reflection 3, 71
self-regulation 91, 102, 119, 123–125
semic method 86, 88, 90, 97
set/*ustanovka* (Uznadze) 11, 29, 50, 130–139, 148–149, 151, 166
Sève, Lucien 149
sexuality 9, 12, 31, 33, 54, 60–63, 67; homosexuality 61–62; libido 10, 62–63, 166; Oedipus complex 10, 55, 67, 150
Sherozia, Apollon 74, 133, 151–153, 155–157
Shevrin, Howard 155
Shmidt, Otto 70
shock therapy 77
Shoshin, P. B. 141, 157
Shuster, Aaron 62
Shvartz, L. 35
Sirotkina, I. 43
slips of the tongue 16, 31, 63, 94, 102, 147, 151, 155
sluggish schizophrenia 96, 99
Smirnov, Anatolii 112, 114–115
Snezhnevsky, Andrei 54, 74

Solms, M. 107
*Sovetskaia iskusstvo* 67–68
*Sovetskaia kul'tura* 65
*Soviet Review* 142
Soviet unconscious 129–161
*Speech and The Development of Mental Processes of the Child* (Luria, 1956) 120
Spielrein, Sabina 25, 27, 32, 60, 84
splitting 20–21, 41, 46, 48, 64, 147
Stalin, Joseph 20, 25–26, 28, 34, 36–40, 42–43, 50, 61–62, 68, 84, 95
Stalinism 2, 17, 20–21, 34, 37, 51, 75, 77, 83, 95, 105, 125
structuralism 158, 160
super-ego 53, 123–125, 130
Symposium on the Unconscious (1979) 4, 10, 63, 74, 93, 103, 129, 138–139, 141–142, 150–158, 161

talking cure 110, 125, 143, 149
Tausk, Victor 25, 31, 66
Tbilisi State University 111, 115
terminology 29, 36–43, *see also* language
*Theories of Personality in Foreign Psychology* (Zeigarnik, 1982) 93
Theory of Functional Systems 6
*Theory of Personality of K. Lewin* (Zeigarnik, 1981) 93–94
Thinking 8, 24, 36, 43–44, 57, 71, 76, 84, 86, 88, 90–93, 93–100, 102–104, 113–114, 123–124, 131, 137, 150, 152, 156
Third Five-Year Plan 40
*Three Essays on the Theory of Sexuality* (Freud, 1924) 155
Tolstoy, Leo 31, 44, 68
*Totem and Taboo* (Freud, 1913) 69
*Traumatic Aphasia* (Luria, 1970) 91
traumatic repetition 82
Trotsky, Leon 25–26, 28
Trotskyism 68
Trubetzkoy, Nikolay 114
Tsaregorodtsev, G. I. 160
twins 120–123

unconscious, Soviet 129–161
*Unconscious, The* (Freud, 1915) 87, 98, 151
*ustanovka see* set/*ustanovka* (Uznadze)
Uznadze, Dmitry 3–4, 6–9, 11, 13, 16–17, 46, 51, 53, 57, 73, 75, 77, 129–139, 141, 147–148, 153–154, 161, 165–166; *Psychology of Set, The* (1966) 132; set/*ustanovka* 11, 29, 50, 130–139, 148–149, 151, 166

Valabrega, Jean Paul 154
van der Veer, R. 86
Varga, Eugen 25
vicissitudes 56, 60, 125, 129, 135, 166
Vnukov, V. 35
Volodin, S. 66
von Brücke, Ernst Wilhelm 54
*Voprosy Filosofi* 52, 129, 159–160
*Voprosy Psikhologii* 93, 129, 131–132, 160
Vrubel, Dmitri 40
Vygotsky, Lev 3, 7, 9, 12, 24, 27–29, 32, 49, 57, 66, 81–88, 95, 97, 105, 112–113, 116, 118–119, 165; banning of 24; birthplace of 7; classification of objects 99; history of 84–85; influence on Zeigarnik 86–88; on schizophrenia 81, 87–88, 100, 139; semic method 86, 88, 90, 97
Vyrgioti, M. 12
Vyrubov, Nikolay 25, 30

Waterlow, Jonathan 15, 20, 44, 47
Weiner, Nobert 53
Weiskopf, Mikhail 39
Winnicott, Donald 81
Wolf Man 98
women 61–62, 83
Wortis, Joseph 52–53
Wulff, Moshe 25, 30

Yaroshevsky, Mikhail 88
Yasnitsky, A. 24, 50, 55, 83, 129
Yeltsin, Boris 36, 150
Yurchak, A. 17–20, 44, 47, 64, 144–145, 160–161

Zajicek, Benjamin 76, 95
Zalkind, Aron B. 60, 63, 67, 112
Zavershneva, E. 86
Zeigarnik, Andrei 83, 85
Zeigarnik, Bluma 4, 6–9, 13, 16, 38, 46, 57, 77, 81–105, 118–119, 123, 125, 131, 137, 139, 149, 159, 165–166; birthplace of 7; *Disturbances of Thinking of Psychiatric Patients* (1958) 96; early years 85; *Experimental Abnormal Psychology* (1972) 93;

*Foundations of Psychopathology* (1973) 92; history of 82–83; husband accused of espionage 83, 89; *Introduction to Pathopsychology* (1969) 82, 92–94, 119; later career 91–93; Luria's co-operation 88–91; *Pathology of Thinking* (1962) 96–97; pathopsychological experiment 81–82, 88, 94, 97, 101, 105, 119; *Personality and Pathology of Activity* (1971) 92; principles of pathopsychology 100–105; reading Freud 93–95; on schizophrenia 81–82, 92, 94–104; and Soviet psychology 83–95; *Theories of Personality in Foreign Psychology* (1982) 93; *Theory of Personality of K. Lewin* (1981) 93–94; Vygotsky's influence 86–88

Zeigarnik effect 82, 86, 143
zone of proximal development 86

For Product Safety Concerns and Information please contact our EU
representative GPSR@taylorandfrancis.com
Taylor & Francis Verlag GmbH, Kaufingerstraße 24, 80331 München, Germany

www.ingramcontent.com/pod-product-compliance
Lightning Source LLC
Chambersburg PA
CBHW050536300426
44113CB00012B/2137